Yasuhiro Nosaka

# Sinus Floor Elevation: Avoiding pitfalls using cone-beam CT

Yasuhiro Nosaka

# Sinus Floor Elevation:

## Avoiding pitfalls using cone-beam CT

QUINTESSENCE PUBLISHING

London, Berlin, Chicago, Tokyo, Barcelona, Beijing, Bucharest, Istanbul, Milan, Moscow, New Delhi, Paris, Prague, Riyadh, São Paulo, Seoul, Singapore, Warsaw and Zagreb

Title of the original edition:
"Pitfalls of Sinus Floor Elevation Verified by Cone-beam CT"


A CIP record for this book is available from the British Library.
ISBN: 978-1-85097-265-5

QUINTESSENCE PUBLISHING

Quintessence Publishing Co. Ltd,
Grafton Road, New Malden, Surrey KT3 3AB,
United Kingdom
www.quintpub.co.uk


Editing: Quintessence Publishing Co. Ltd, London, UK
Layout and Production: Janina Kuhn, Quintessenz Verlags-GmbH, Berlin, Germany

Printed and bound in Germany

# Foreword

The maxillary sinus is very small in infancy and early childhood, and it grows with the process of tooth eruption, and thus a large pneumatic cavity is formed between the orbital foramen and the alveolar ridge.

There are various views as to the function of this cavity. I believe it prevents a direct impact of an apical lesion of a molar (if it develops) on the eyes. If an abscess develops in the apical region, purulent discharge through the ostium protects the orbital foramen from being affected. I feel it is a rational assumption that the maxillary sinus grows in size to serve as a protective barrier for the eyes. In a dog, only a small sinus cavity exists right under the orbital foramen. In humans, however, a very large cavity is present under the orbital foramen to maintain the balance between the large brain and the small jaw.

When a tooth is lost, the alveolar bone supporting the tooth undergoes disuse resorption. Through this process, the maxillary sinus becomes a structure just like an eggshell with aging. Sinus floor elevation by the lateral window or osteotome techniques is a procedure to reduce the cavity size to facilitate implant placements. The maxillary sinus is in the process of forming an eggshell-like structure, and sinus floor elevation is surgery completely counter to the body's process. Should the surgery fail, therefore, significant damage is unavoidable. It should also be noted that failure of the surgery can lead to less confidence in the reliability of dental implants and the abilities of oral surgeons.

While recognizing the benefit of less invasiveness, Dr Yasuhiro Nosaka has pointed out in this book some drawbacks of the osteotome technique, such as the difficulty of judging success or failure due to the blindness of the surgery, and less assurance of implant functioning. Actual examples of implant dislocation into the sinus cavity, including the difficulties of removing dislocated implants, are presented. To resolve such a problem promptly, it is important to maintain good collaboration between general practitioners and oral surgery facilities.

In this book, the author recommends performing thorough preoperative examinations by means of CT imaging for dental use (3DX, Morita, Japan) and the use of a fiberscope; and, if any problem is detected, not providing sinus floor elevation until the problem is properly treated. This book presents details, including pathological findings of manifold cases, such as the treatment of maxillary sinusitis, mucous retention cysts and apical lesions, as well as solutions for cases with difficulties due to the presence of alveolar artery and septa.

Of special note is the description on the use of titanium mesh over lateral windows, and the elucidation of the process of bone regeneration up to maturation in the form of cortical and cancellous bone – both evidenced by long-term observation. This book shows us the whole story of the reappearance of once-lost alveolar bone.

The only way to ensure good outcomes is to avoid "pitfalls" through careful evaluations and diagnosis. I strongly believe that the author is always trying to learn from every failure and not to repeat the same mistakes. I hope this book will become a guide for readers in achieving more reliable and safe implant treatments.

*Yoshinori Arai*
Professor, Nihon University Dental School
(developer of cone-beam CT for dental use)
August 2010

# Preface

Dental implants are now seen as an established treatment modality. Despite our growing knowledge and experiences, however, much about implant treatment remains unknown. Biological processes and mechanisms relating to sinus floor elevation, in particular, have yet to be fully elucidated, and any uncertainties about surgical procedures and grafting materials may result in unwanted treatment outcomes. Conventional postoperative evaluation by panoramic radiographs provides only two-dimensional information and may not be good enough to precisely evaluate the outcomes of sinus floor elevation. Pathological specimens are also limited in terms of the target area and timing and may not be able to provide convincing information about the prognosis of sinus floor elevation.

I experienced sinus floor elevation for the first time under the mentorship of Professor Minoru Ueda of Nagoya University, about 15 years ago. Since then, I have provided about 250 sinus floor elevation surgeries in various hospitals and clinics. The postoperative outcomes of these surgeries were evaluated, mainly based on panoramic radiographs and short-term clinical results.

It was cone-beam computed tomography (CBCT) that brought about significant changes in my clinical attitude. Cone-beam CT produces clear images (in spite of an extremely low radiation dose), so it can be a very useful tool for pre- and postoperative evaluation of sinus floor elevation procedures. Longitudinal follow-up of each patient also facilitates precise evaluation of the biological reaction of the surgical site. The model 3DX (Morita, Japan) we have in our clinic can scan an area of 6 cm × 6 cm, which is considered to be the minimum necessary for sinus floor evaluation. This small scan area can also assure the minimum radiation exposure, which is one of the most important benefits of CBCT. The image is clear enough for monitoring the changes in trabecular bone, and thus allows evaluation of bone modeling and remodeling.

This book has two sections, covering sinus floor elevations by the lateral window and osteotome techniques. The pre- and postoperative evaluations by CBCT are analyzed to make clear the pitfalls (or traps) to which we are prone. The new findings or the facts revealed by CBCT scanning are also presented for further discussion, for more predictable procedures and grafting materials.

The author believes that we cannot be confident about the safety of a surgical procedure unless we have in-depth detailed postoperative evaluations of at least 50 cases treated by the procedure. We have to keep the saying "body response seldom lies" firmly in mind when we provide dental implant treatments. What we as dentists can do is guide, not control, the body's response. A solid understanding of body reaction is of extreme importance, and I hope you will find something of value in this book in improving your understanding of the biological response to sinus floor elevation.

On a final note, we are all indebted to patients who provide us with a lot of new important findings. Also, special thanks to Professor Yoshinori Arai who developed CBCT for dental use and realized the model 3DX.

*Yasuhiro Nosaka*

July, 2010

# Acknowledgments

This book would not have been possible without the support of many people.

The author wishes to express his gratitude for their support and guidance to: Dr Kazuhiko Hamamoto, who is the director of Hamamoto Dentistry and Oral Surgery Clinic; Dr Tatsuya Kawamura, who is the director of Osaka Implant & Regenerative Medical Center; and Dr Hitomi Nosaka, who is the author's dearest wife and a dentist of Nosaka Oral Surgery Clinic.

The author would also like to give special thanks to all the staff of Nosaka Oral Surgery Clinic: Ms Nao Hirata, dental hygienist; Ms Mio Sato, dental hygienist; Ms Michie Murase, receptionist; and Ms Miho Ichikawa and Ms Atsuko Hisayama, dental assistants.

# Author

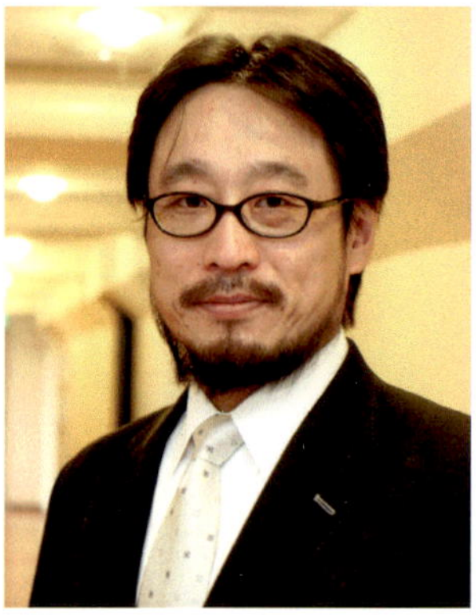


## Yasuhiro Nosaka, DDS, PhD

Director, Nosaka Oral Surgery Clinic
Email: nosasen@aol.com


DDS, Osaka Dental University
PhD, Osaka Dental University Graduate School

| | |
|---|---|
| 1991 | Head oral surgeon, Nissay Hospital |
| 1995 | Lecturer, Oral Surgery Dept., Nagoya University School of Medicine |
| 1997 | Visiting lecturer, Oral Surgery Dept., Osaka Dental University |
| 1999 | Visiting lecturer, Kobe University School of Medicine |
| 2000 | Head oral surgeon, Kobe City Medical Center West Hospital |
| 2005 | Director, Nosaka Oral Surgery Clinic |
| 2009 | Committee member, The Japanese Society of Oral Implantology |
| | Committee member, The Japanese Society of Regenerative Medicine |

## Bibliography


Nosaka Y, Tsunokuma M, Hayashi H, Kakudo K. Placement of osseointegrated implants in distraction osteogenesis: A pilot study in dogs. Int J Oral Maxillofac Implants 2000;15:185–192.

Nosaka Y. Placement of implants into distracted bone: Craniofacial distraction osteogenesis. USA: Mosby, 2001:62–67.

Nosaka Y, Tachi Y, Shimpuku H, Kawamura T, Ohura K. Association of calcitonin receptor gene polymorphism with early marginal bone loss around endosseous implants. Int J Oral Maxillofac Implants 2002;17:38–43.

Nosaka Y, Kitano S, Wada K, Komori T. Endossesous implants in horizontal alveolar ridge distraction osteogenesis. Int J Oral Maxillofac Implants 2002;17:846–853.

Nosaka Y, Kobayashi M, Kitano S, Komori T. Horizontal alveolar ridge distraction osteogenesis in dogs: radiographic and histologic studies. Int J Oral Maxillofac Implants 2005;20:837–842.

# Contents

# PART 1 The lateral window technique aided by CT scanning

# CHAPTER 1

# The maxillary sinus and membrane

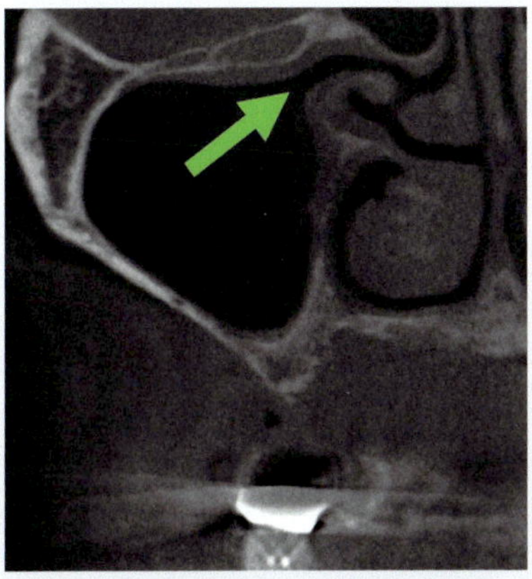

**Fig 1-1** Transverse section of a cone-beam CT scan showing the ostium and connection to the nasal cavity.

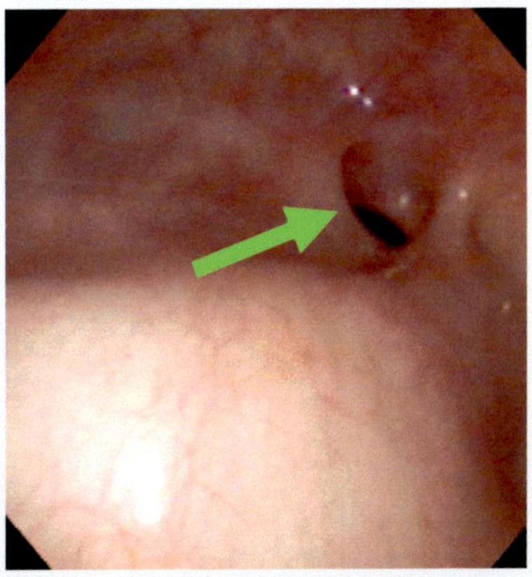

**Fig 1-2** Ostium viewed from the maxillary sinus cavity.

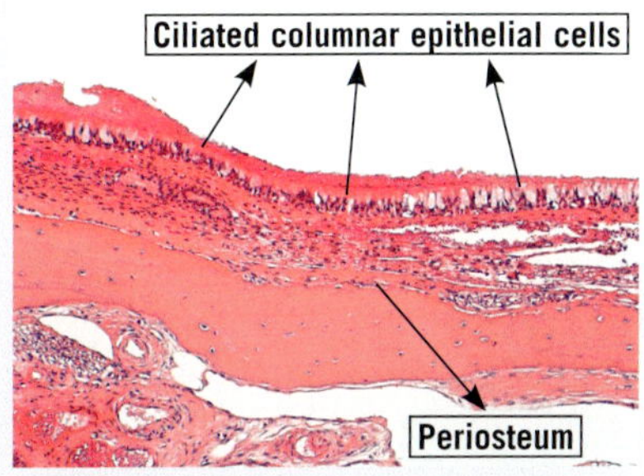


**Fig 1-3** Bone and sinus membrane harvested from the anterior wall of the maxillary sinus (HE-staining).

## Role of the maxillary sinus membrane in excretion of foreign substances

The maxillary sinus, located in the body of the maxilla, is the largest of the paranasal sinuses. It communicates with the nasal cavity through the ostium (green arrow on Fig 1-1), through which the air flows into and out of the maxillary sinus during expiration and inspiration, respectively (green arrow on Fig 1-2). The role of the maxillary sinus membrane is to remove airborne substances such as dust, microorganisms or pollen introduced into the maxillary sinus during expiration.

The maxillary sinus membrane contains ciliated columnar epithelial cells, and their ciliary movements work to keep the maxillary sinus clean by removing foreign substances out through the ostium (Fig 1-3).

## Maxillary empyema

The disorder involving accumulation of pus and foreign substances within the maxillary sinus arising from ciliary motility dysfunction of the membrane is generally termed "maxillary empyema". The maxillary sinus membrane has periosteum on the osseous side, but it is not as strong as that of the mandibular bone and is easily perforated during membrane elevation.

> **! Key Point**
>
> Although the maxillary sinus membrane has periosteum on the osseous side, it is not as strong as that on the mandibular bone and is easily perforated during membrane elevation.

## Informed consent

Sinus floor elevation requires a full understanding of the anatomy and physiology of the maxillary sinus. For informed consent, patients must be given sufficient information on the treatment procedure and expected benefits and risks, including the likelihood of each benefit and risk. Making a self-serving assumption that the patient will not be able to understand an explanation could be an invitation to serious trouble. In the author's clinic, all candidates for a sinus floor elevation procedure are given explanations of the anatomy and physiology of the maxillary sinus. Most patients find this relatively easy to understand (in Japan, partly due to the fact that the term "maxillary empyema" is quite well known).

# CHAPTER 2

# CT scanning for maxillary sinus evaluation

Only CT scanning can properly evaluate the maxillary sinus. Panoramic radiography is insufficient for accurate examination and evaluation of maxillary sinus morphologies or lesions. In particular, accurate evaluation of lesions of the maxillary sinus mucosa is impossible without CT scanning.

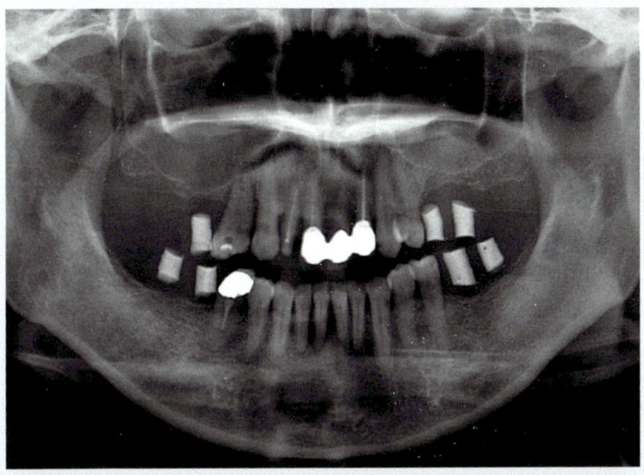

**Fig 2-1** Panoramic view: evidence of mucosal swelling in the maxillary sinus floor only on the left side.

## Blind spot 1: Maxillary sinusitis cannot be diagnosed by panoramic radiography

This patient was referred for CT examination prior to implant placements in both sides of the posterior maxilla and mandible. Though not found on the panoramic radiograph (Fig 2-1), swelling of the maxillary sinus mucosa on the right side was apparent on CT scans (Figs 2-2 and 2-3). The swelling was severe with no pneumatic space remaining. Mucosal swelling on the left side, which had been expected from the contrast difference between the mucosa and the air sinus on the panoramic radiograph, was also confirmed by CT images (Figs 2-4 and 2-5).

Before implant placement, sinus floor elevation by means of the lateral window technique was considered necessary after treatment of the right and left maxillary sinusitis.

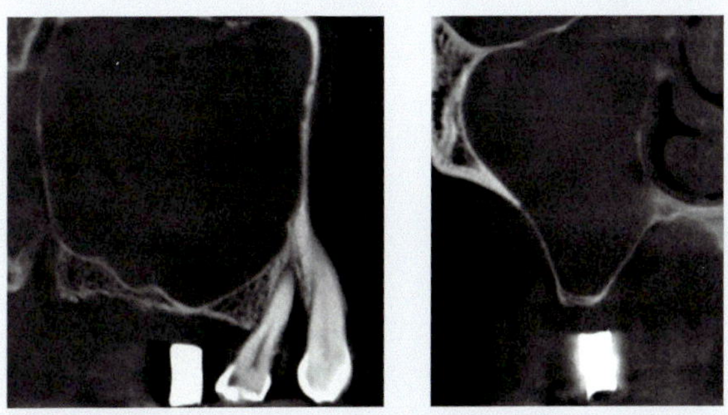

**Figs 2-2 and 2-3** Swelling of the maxillary sinus mucosa on the right side.

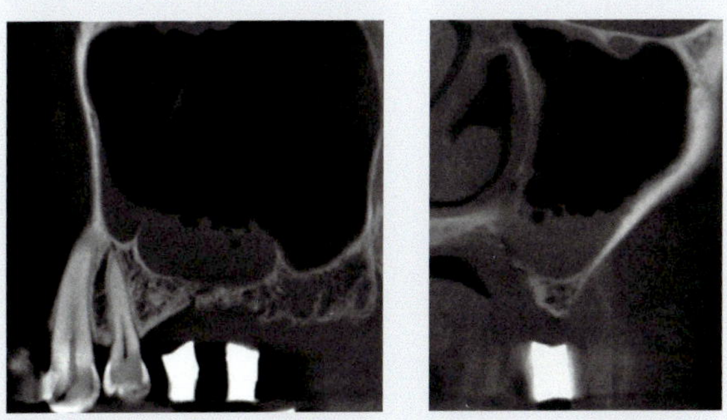

**Figs 2-4 and 2-5** Mucosal swelling on the left side.

## Blind spot 2: Cause of a fistula determined by CT scan

In this patient there was no problem with the gingiva around teeth 17 and 16. A fistula was found at 15. The cause of the fistula could not be identified on a panoramic radiograph.

The patient was referred for two reasons: (i) a fistula located at region 15 (black arrow on Fig 2-6) despite the fact that tooth 15 was missing; and (ii) dome-shaped radiopacity (yellow arrows on Fig 2-7) on the panoramic radiograph. A sagittal CT

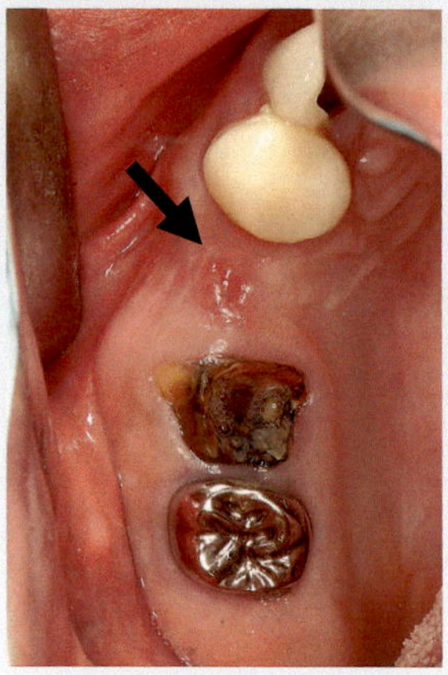

Fig 2-6 (left) Intraoral view.

Fig 2-7 (right) Panoramic view.

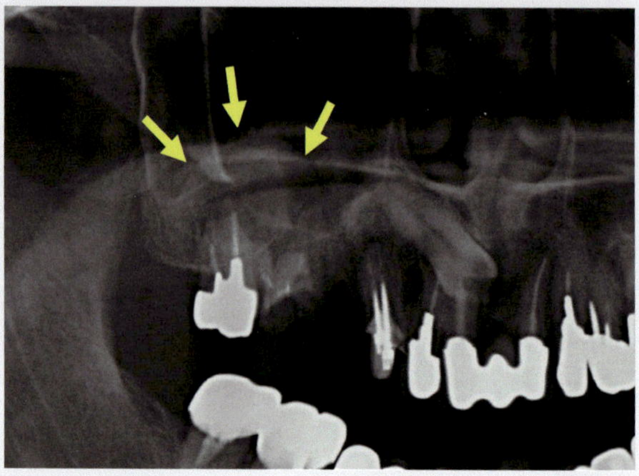

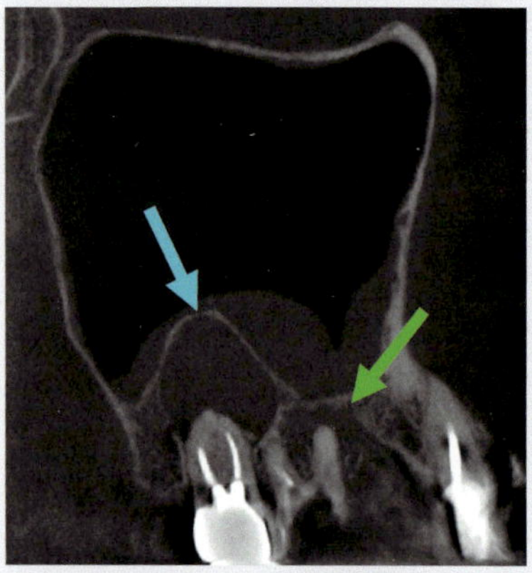

Fig 2-8 Sagittal CT image.

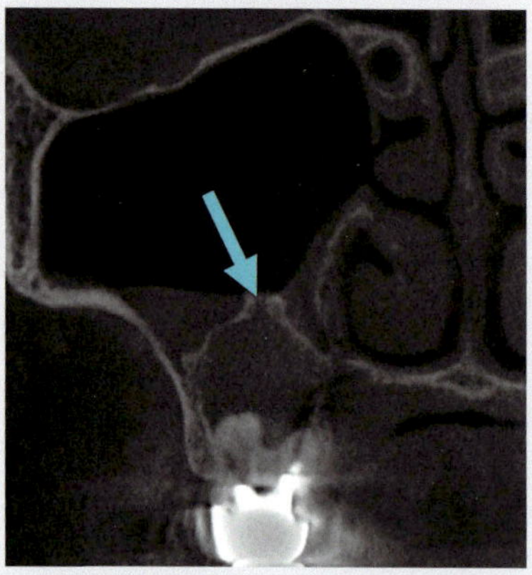

Fig 2-9 Buccolingual CT image at tooth 17.

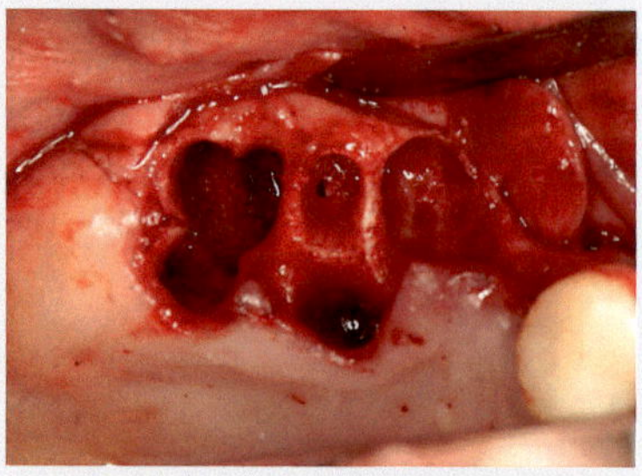

Fig 2-10 Situation after removal of the cyst. A comparatively large cyst on the mesiobuccal root of tooth 16 seemed to be the cause of the fistula.

scan showed cyst-like radiolucency at the mesial root of tooth 16 (green arrow on Fig 2-8) and at the apex of tooth 17 (blue arrows on Figs 2-8 and 2-9), and the fistula seemed to have been caused by the cyst at the mesiobuccal root of tooth 16. There was a bony layer above the cyst at tooth 17. However, the maxillary sinus membrane at tooth 17 exhibited swelling, which indicated that the bony layer did not function as a barrier against the spread of inflammation.

Teeth 16 and 17 were extracted and the cyst was removed. No perforation of the maxillary sinus membrane was found (Fig 2-10).

**! Key Point**

CT imaging made it possible to determine that the fistula was caused by the cyst at the mesiobuccal root of tooth 16.

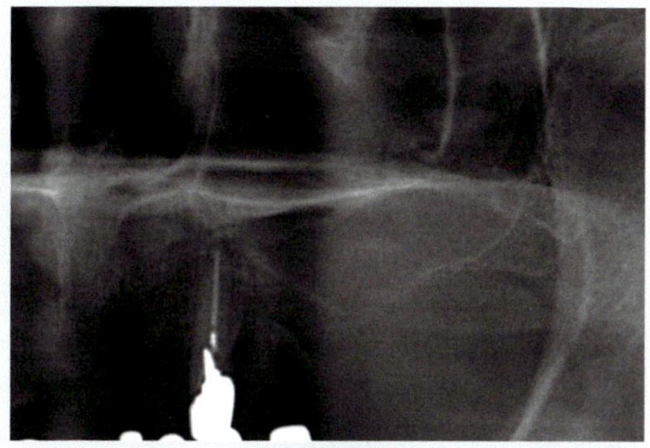

**Fig 2-11** Panoramic radiograph showing a dome-shaped radiopacity.

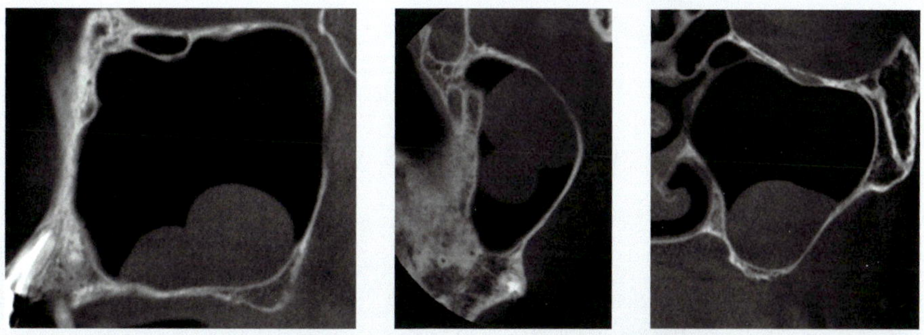

**Figs 2-12 to 2-14** CT imaging reveals dome-shaped radiopacity at two locations, and no swelling of the maxillary sinus mucous outside the lesion.

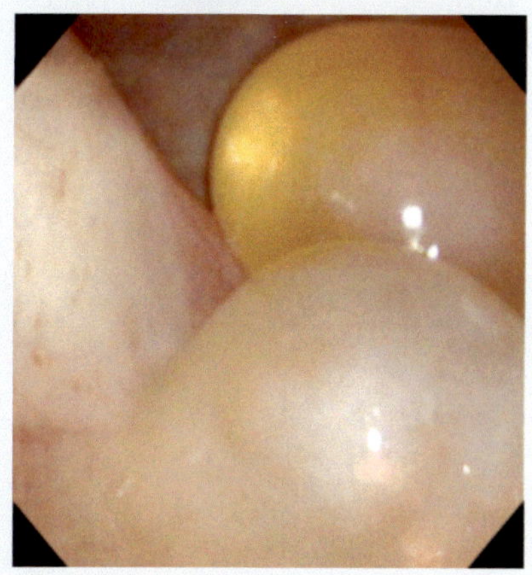

**Fig 2-15** A cyst containing clear yellowish fluid was detected by a fiberscope and diagnosed as a mucous retention cyst.

## Blind spot 3: Diagnosis of a mucous retention cyst by CT scanning

This patient was referred for a sinus floor elevation on the left side by the lateral window technique. A panoramic radiograph showed a dome-shaped radiopacity but could not provide information on the three-dimensional location and the condition of the maxillary sinus membrane outside the lesion (Fig 2-11). CT imaging revealed dome-shaped radiopacity at two locations, and no swelling of the maxillary sinus mucous outside the lesion (Figs 2-12 to 2-14). A fiberscope inserted through the canine fossa found two cysts containing clear yellowish fluid, diagnosed as mucous retention cysts (Fig 2-15). It should be noted that CT is not capable of evaluating the fluid contained within the cyst.

**! Key Point**

CT imaging is incapable of evaluating the nature of the fluid contained within a cyst.

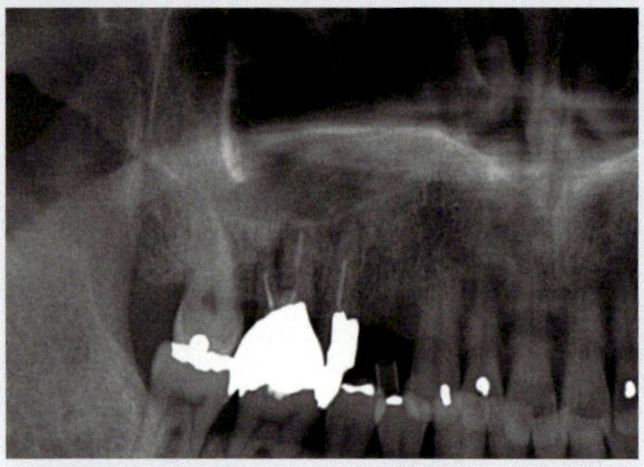

**Fig 2-16** Panoramic view of the odontogenic lesion.

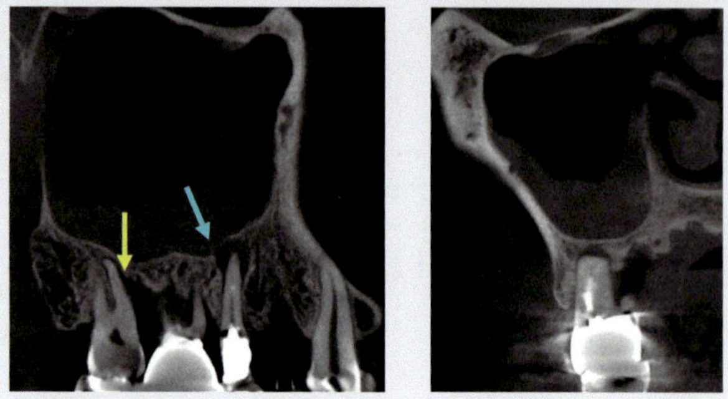

**Figs 2-17 and 2-18** CT imaging reveals further information on the defects.

## Blind spot 4: Maxillary sinus membrane swelling of odontogenic origin confirmed by CT scanning

This patient was referred for preoperative examination prior to implant placement at region 14. Although it was not clear on the panoramic radiograph (Fig 2-16), CT scanning revealed bone resorption up to the tooth apex at the mesiobuccal root of tooth 17 (yellow arrow on Fig 2-17) and swelling of the maxillary sinus membrane (Figs 2-17 and 2-18). Furthermore, a cyst-like radiolucency was seen at the apex of tooth 15, where a defect of cortical bone of the maxillary sinus floor was found (blue arrow on Fig 2-17).

> **! Key Point**
>
> There was a cyst-like radiolucency at the apex of tooth 15, where a cortical bone defect of the maxillary sinus floor was found.

## Blind spot 5: Septum shape cannot be seen on a panoramic radiograph

This patient was referred for preoperative examination prior to sinus augmentation on the right side by the lateral window technique. A panoramic radiograph showed irregular radiopacity at the regions of teeth 17 and 16 (yellow arrow on Fig 2-19). CT scanning revealed that this irregular radiopacity resulted from the fusion of two septa (Figs 2-20 to 2-23). Sinus floor elevation at this location was considered to be fairly difficult.

> **! Key Point**
>
> CT scanning revealed the fusion of two septa. Sinus membrane elevation at this location is considered to be fairly difficult.

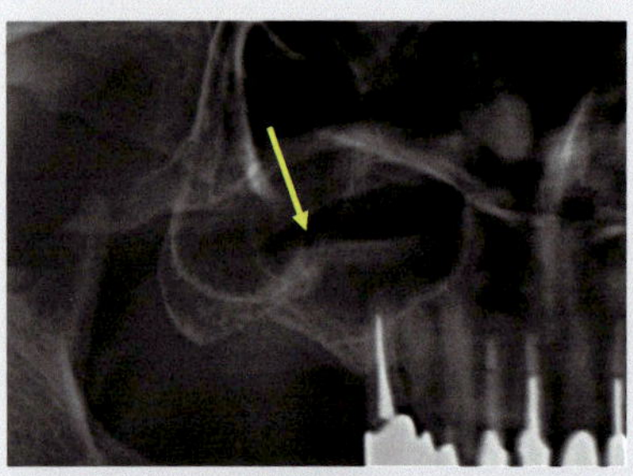

**Fig 2-19** Panoramic view.

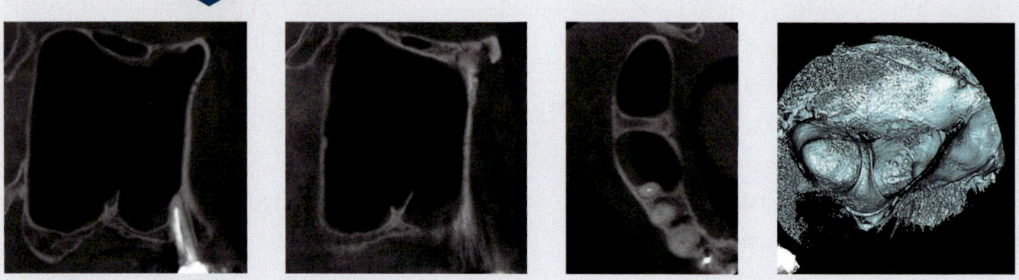

**Figs 2-20 to 2-23** CT imaging reveals a fusion of two septa. The CT slices should be chosen in various directions.

CHAPTER 3

# Principles and procedures of the lateral window technique

## Introduction

The lateral window technique is used to facilitate the placement of endosteal implants of sufficient length in patients with limited osseous height in the posterior maxilla, due to excessive downward growth of the maxillary sinus (pink arrows on Fig 3-1).

Osteotomy of the anterior wall of the maxillary sinus is performed with careful attention to prevent sinus membrane perforation. Through the opening made during the procedure, the sinus membrane is dissected from the bony walls and elevated. The bone block made by the osteotomy is called a **lateral window** or **trapdoor** (yellow arrow on Fig 3-2).

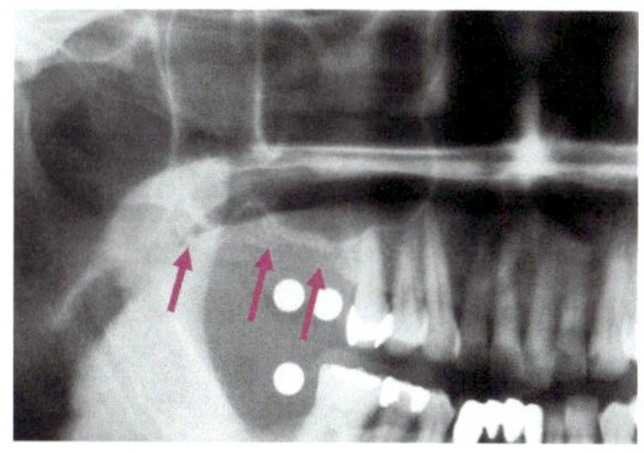

**Fig 3-1** Limited osseous height in the posterior maxilla.

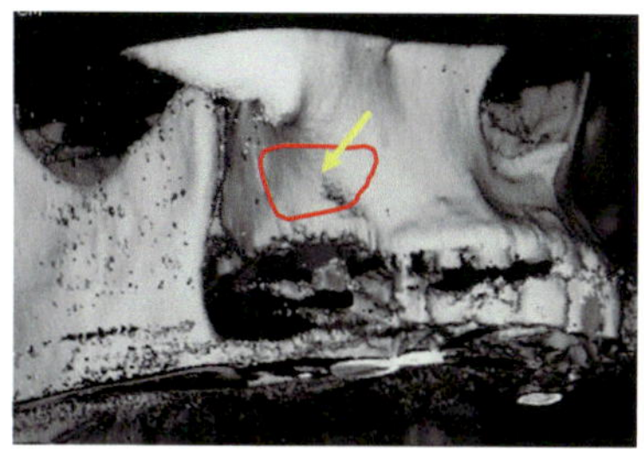

**Fig 3-2** The lateral window.

## Surgical procedure

After reflecting a mucoperiosteal flap, a lateral window is created on the maxillary sinus anterior wall by osteotomy using a round diamond bur (blue arrows on Fig 3-3). Extreme caution is required to prevent perforation of the sinus membrane during the osteotomy. The yellow line and the red areas on the helical CT image indicate the sinus membrane and the osteotomy areas, respectively (Fig 3-4).

After completion of the osteotomy, the sinus membrane at the margin of the lateral window is dissected and then elevated superiorly by gently pushing the lateral window into the sinus cavity. Eventually the sinus membrane on the medial wall is fully detached (purple arrows on Figs 3-5 and 3-6), and both the lateral window and the sinus membrane are pushed upward (Figs 3-5 and 3-6). The empty compartment created by elevating the sinus membrane is filled with grafting material and allowed to heal. After there has been new bone formation to gain adequate bone height, the implant of appropriate length is inserted.Simultaneous implant placement with sinus floor elevation can be an option if good primary stability of the implant is achieved.

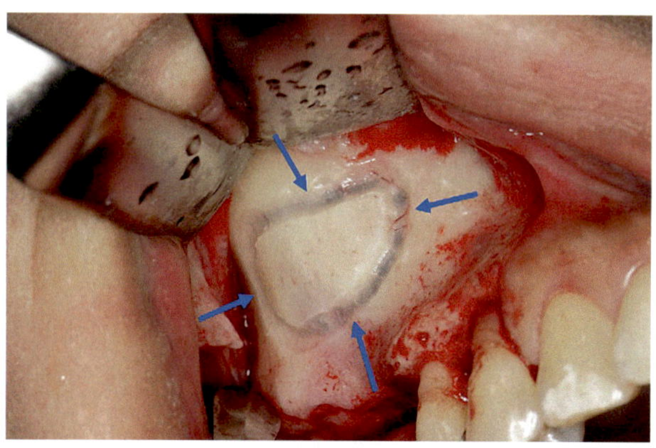

**Fig 3-3** Starting the osteotomy.

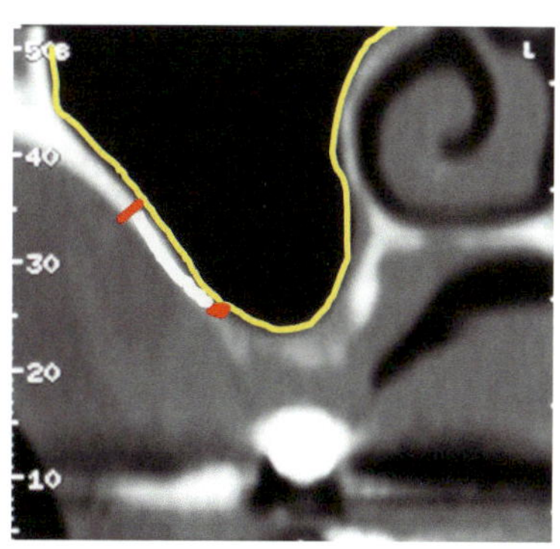


**Fig 3-4** CT of the sinus membrane and the osteotomy areas.

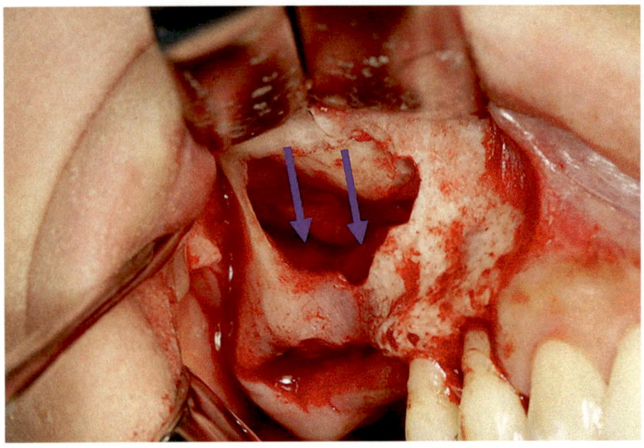

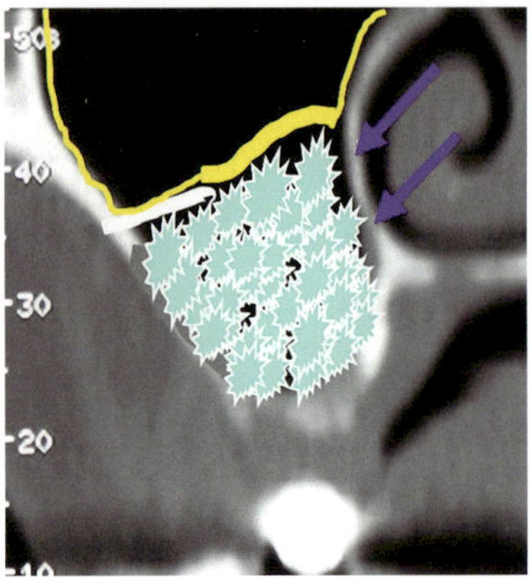


**Fig 3-5** (left) Detaching the sinus membrane on the medial wall.

**Fig 3-6** (right) CT after the lateral window and the sinus membrane have been pushed upward.

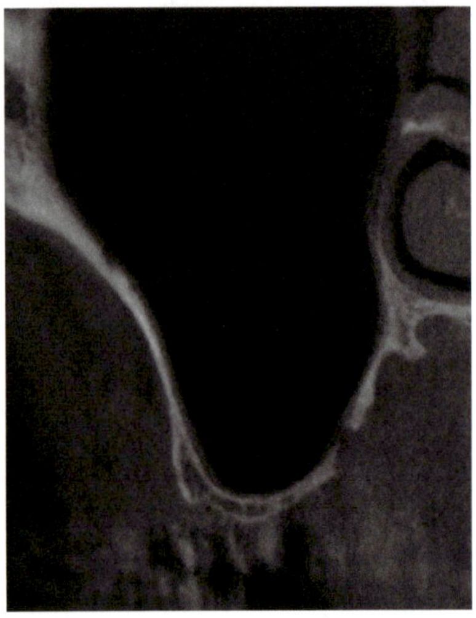

**Fig 3-7** Preoperative CT image.

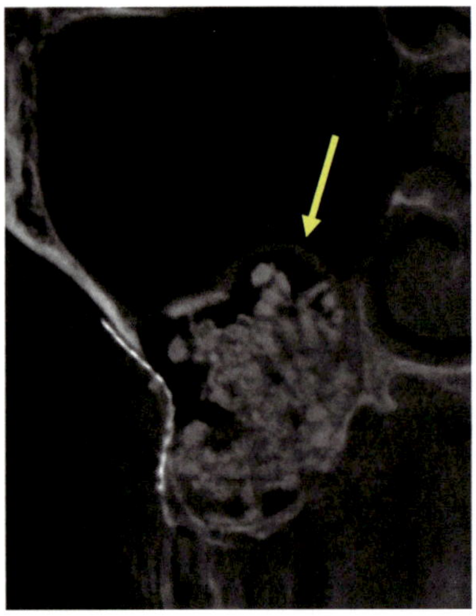

**Fig 3-8** CT image immediately after surgery.

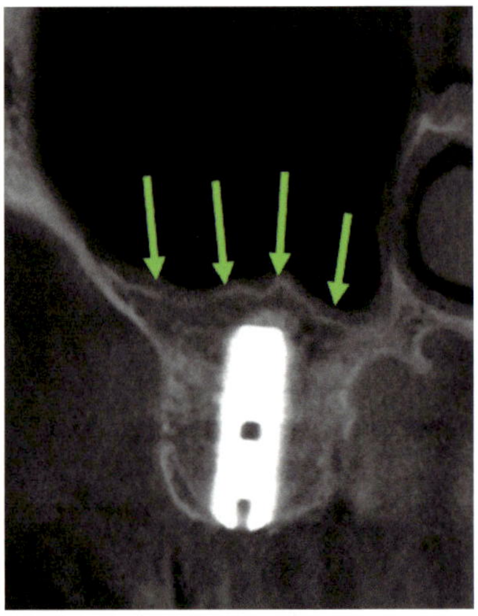

**Fig 3-9** CT image after 1 year.

## Contraction and thickening of a detached sinus membrane

Conventional postoperative evaluation of the lateral window technique includes many factors that remain presumptive, and in reality often turns out to be very different. This highlights the importance of postoperative evaluation and verification by CT imaging.

Schema describing sinus floor elevation procedures often employ wave-like lines to represent elevated sinus membranes. However, there is no such finding on an actual postoperative CT image. An intact maxillary sinus membrane cannot be observed on a preoperative CT scan, but a CT image taken immediately after sinus floor elevation shows the elevated membrane as a radiopaque line (Fig 3-7, yellow arrow on Fig 3-8). The lateral window is covered with a titanium mesh plate.

The detached sinus membrane contracts and becomes thicker, which is considered to contribute to the appearance of the radiopaque line on a CT image.

One year after the surgery, the cortical-like bone is observed at the newly formed bottom of the maxillary sinus as the radiopaque line (green arrows on Fig 3-9).

## Bone graft materials

Grafting materials available today are divided into two main categories: autogenous bone grafts and synthetic bone substitutes. Bone substitutes are further classified into resorbable and nonresorbable types.

The author uses beta-tricalcium phosphate (β-TCP), which resorbs and is replaced by bone tissue. However, a small amount of β-TCP granules still remain 12 months following implantation, and the mechanical strength of the augmented bone is comparable to that of foamed polystyrene. The author makes it a rule to allow the region augmented by β-TCP to heal for 12 months prior to implant placement.

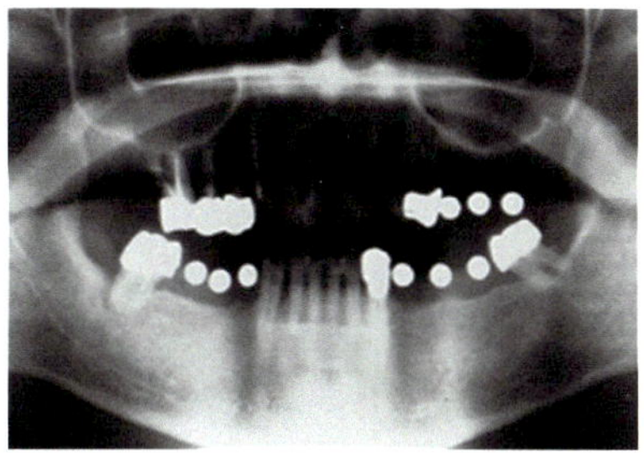

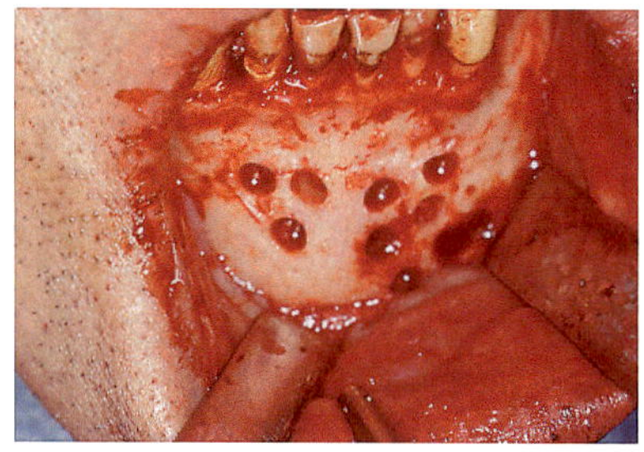

**Fig 3-10** (left) Preoperative panoramic view.

**Fig 3-11** (right) Intraoperative intraoral view.

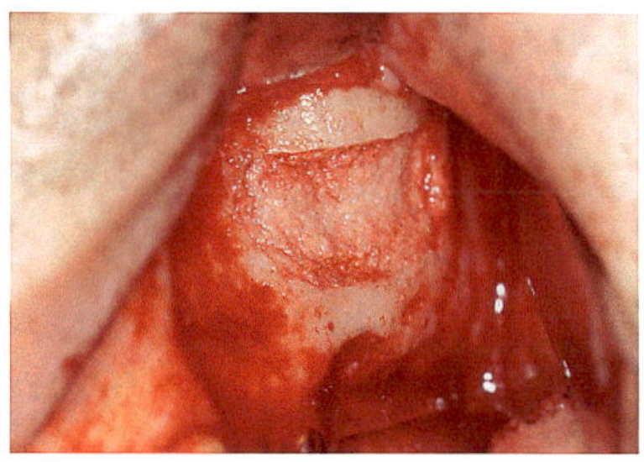

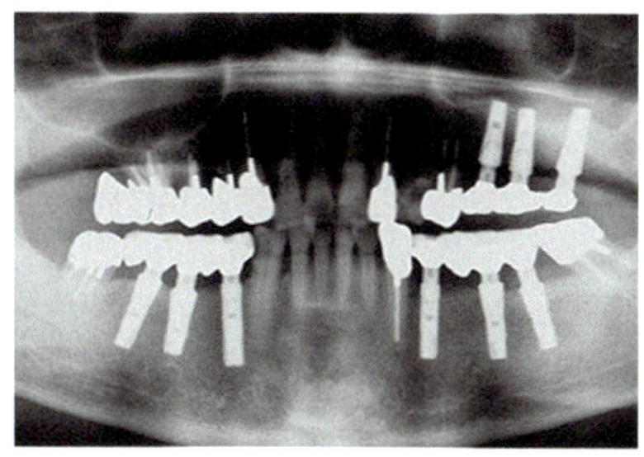

**Fig 3-12** (left) Intraoperative intraoral view.

**Fig 3-13** (right) Postoperative panoramic view.

There are a wide variety of nonresorbable bone substitutes on the market. Currently the author chooses not to use them owing to some concerns about their effectiveness (discussed further in a later section).

> **! Key Point**
>
> A small amount of β-TCP granules remains 12 months after implantation. The mechanical strength of the augmented bone is close to that of foamed polystyrene.

# Issues in harvesting intraoral bone grafts

## General points

Autogenous bone grafts are frequently harvested intraorally, but the surgeon must be aware of the known risks described below:

1. Adequate bone height gained by the lateral window technique requires a substantial amount of grafting material. In many instances, the buccolingual dimension of the maxillary sinus is large and the amount of bone chips harvested intraorally may be insufficient to achieve the desired increase in bone height.
2. Autogenous bone chips are often mixed with bone substitute material to increase the volume, but the optimal mixture ratio and grafting success rates are not fully known. Furthermore, the blood supply to autogenous bone chips may be hindered by the surrounding grafting material, with consequent sequestrum formation. In the author's opinion, the benefits of mixing autogenous bone graft and synthetic bone substitutes are still not fully elucidated.
3. The chin is cited in many books on implant surgery as a donor site where a large volume of autogenous bone can be safely harvested. Nevertheless, harvesting autogenous bone from the chin involves risks, including: (i) postoperative paresthesia in the lower anterior region; (ii) limitation of bone volume available because the donor site is at least 7 mm below the tooth apex; and (iii) marked internal hemorrhage often experienced following surgery in the area from the chin to anterior neck.

## Internal hemorrhage after bone graft harvesting from the chin

For sinus floor elevation by the lateral window technique on the left side, an autogenous bone graft was harvested from a patient's chin using Osteo-Harvestor (OsteoMed; Figs 3-10 to 3-13). This was

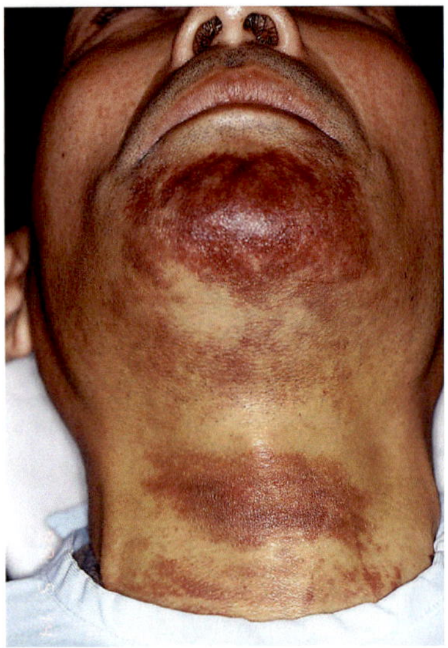

**Fig 3-14** Pronounced internal hemorrhage.

expected to be uneventful, but pronounced internal hemorrhage developed after the surgery in an area extending from the chin to the anterior neck (Fig 3-14).

The author therefore currently employs bone chips harvested from iliac bone marrow for patients who require an autogenous bone graft, and β-TCP for those who require a bone substitute material. In either case, the author uses autogenous bone alone or β-TCP alone, never a combination of the two.

# CHAPTER 4

# Pitfalls of the lateral window technique

This chapter has three parts:

- The preoperative stage
- The intraoperative stage
- The postoperative stage.

## 4.1 The preoperative stage

The lateral window technique is a special bone augmentation operation that is fairly invasive and involves dissection and elevation of the maxillary sinus membrane. If a situation arises that requires a premature ending to the surgery, or any complication such as postoperative infection, the subsequent recovery process is not easy. This surgery is akin to a "one-shot game," so preoperative evaluation is of extreme importance and *any* lesion in the maxillary sinus must be carefully examined by CT analysis.

> **! Key Point**
>
> If any lesion is found in the maxillary sinus, augmentation surgery must not be performed until the lesion has been treated and completely healed. This includes removal of the cause of the lesion.

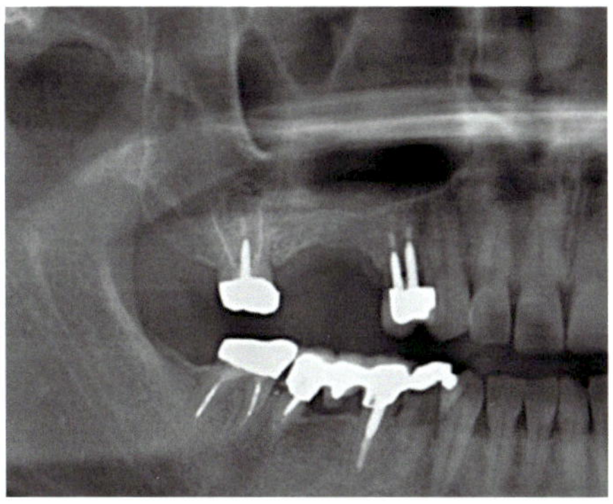

**Fig 4-1** Panoramic view.

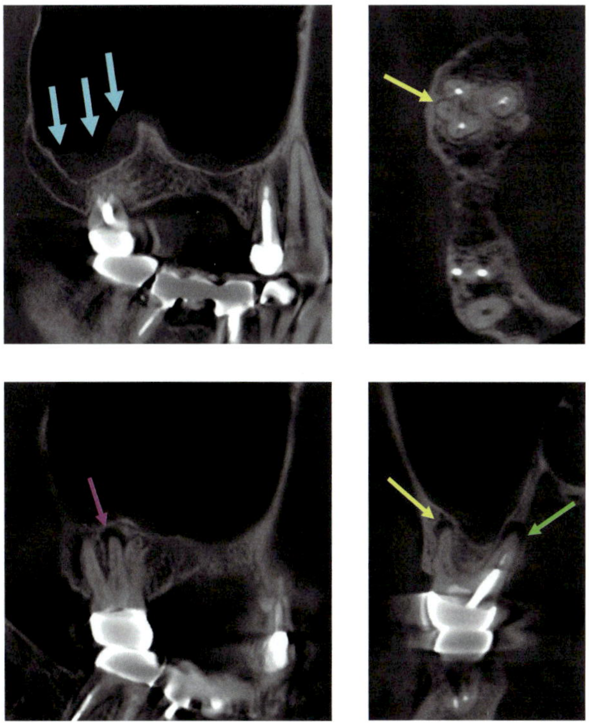

**Figs 4-2 to 4-5** CT images.

### Check point 1: Sinus membrane thickening

In this example, CT scanning revealed swelling of the sinus membrane, an untreated root canal and apical lesion. If sinus floor elevation were to be performed under these conditions, postoperative infection might occur from the lesion of tooth 17.

The patient with loss of teeth 16 and 15 was referred for implant treatment. Downward growth of the maxillary sinus and bone resorption of the alveolar crest revealed by panoramic radiography indicated the need for sinus augmentation by the lateral window technique and guided bone regeneration (GBR; Fig 4-1). A CT scan revealed swelling of the sinus membrane (blue arrows on Fig 4-2), untreated buccal root canal of tooth 17 (yellow arrow on Fig 4-3) and periapical radiolucency (pink arrow on Fig 4-4). There was also another lesion at the palatal root apex (green arrow on Fig 4-5).

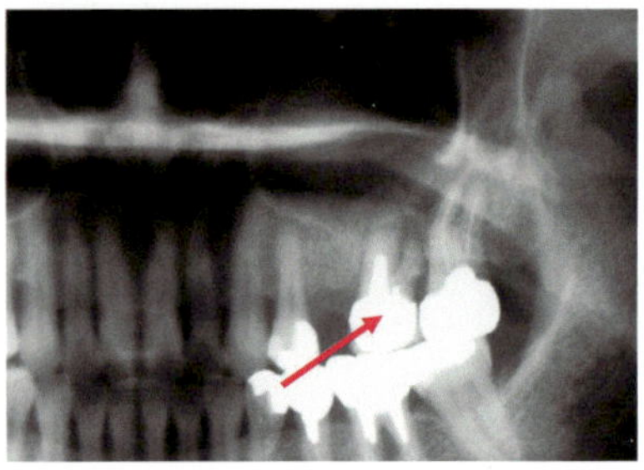

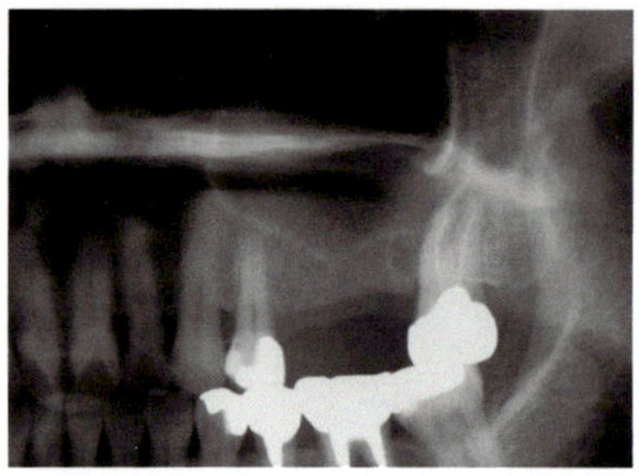

**Fig 4-6** (left) Panoramic view before extraction.

**Fig 4-7** (right) Panoramic view after extraction.

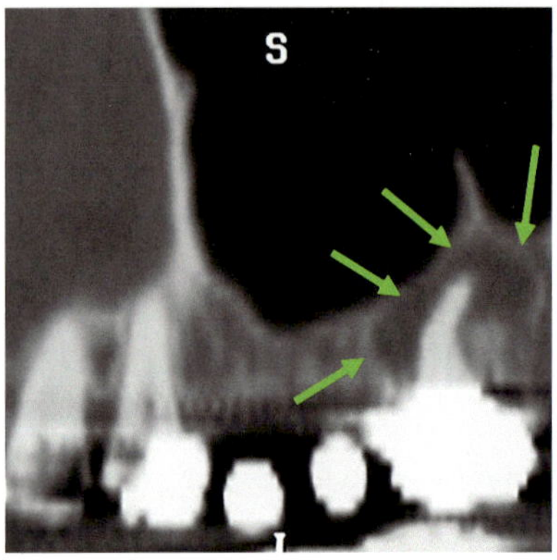


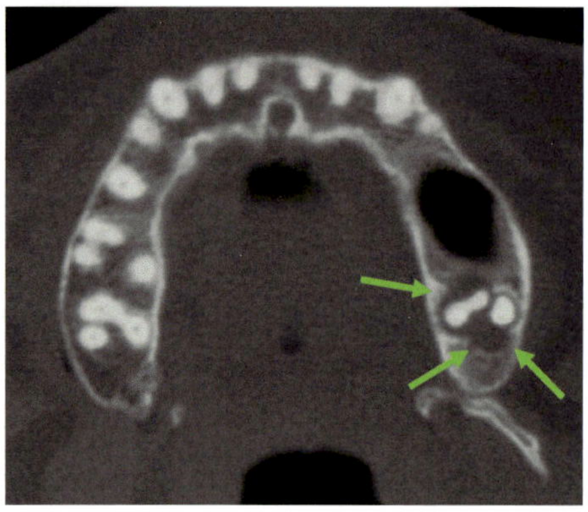

**Figs 4-8 and 4-9** CT images.

The swelling of the sinus membrane was deemed to be secondary inflammation arising from the periapical lesion of tooth 17. Moreover, the thin layer of cortical bone on the sinus floor appeared to be ineffective as a physical barrier against the spread of inflammation. Therefore, if sinus augmentation were to be performed under the present situation, postoperative infection might occur from the lesion at tooth 17.

> **! Key Point**
>
> Root canal therapy of tooth 17 should be provided first. Sinus augmentation surgery should be performed only after the swelling of the sinus membrane has diminished.

## Check point 2: Radicular cyst

This is a case where a patient's radicular cyst was missed because an assessment was based only on panoramic radiography, resulting in a prolonged treatment period.

The patient with loss of tooth 25 was referred for implant treatment. The panoramic radiograph taken by the patient's regular dentist indicated an apical lesion at 26 (Fig 4-6) and the affected tooth had been removed (Fig 4-7). Six months after the extraction, we performed a helical CT scan based on the assumption that sinus augmentation would be necessary for implant placement. Though it was not clear on the original panoramic radiograph, a cyst-like radiolucency (green arrows on Figs 4-8 and 4-9) was detected around tooth 27. CT scanning during the initial examination could have prevented this missed diagnosis.

The patient was sent back to his regular dentist for extraction of tooth 27 and cyst removal. We then treated the patient 6 months after the cyst removal. The treatment period was then shortened through simultaneous sinus floor elevation and implant insertion.

> **! Key Point**
>
> A CT scan taken during initial treatment could have prevented the underdiagnosis. Omission of the CT scan was regrettable.

Shown next are the panoramic radiograph and CT images taken 6 months after the extraction of tooth 27 (Figs 4-10 to 4-14). The residual bone height was approximately 5 mm, which indicated the need for sinus floor elevation. Since 6 months had already been lost, we decided to simultaneously perform the sinus floor elevation and implant placement, provided that good primary stability was achieved. The maxillary sinus of this patient was large in buccolingual width and required a large amount of grafting material. The patient requested that we use bone substitute material alone.

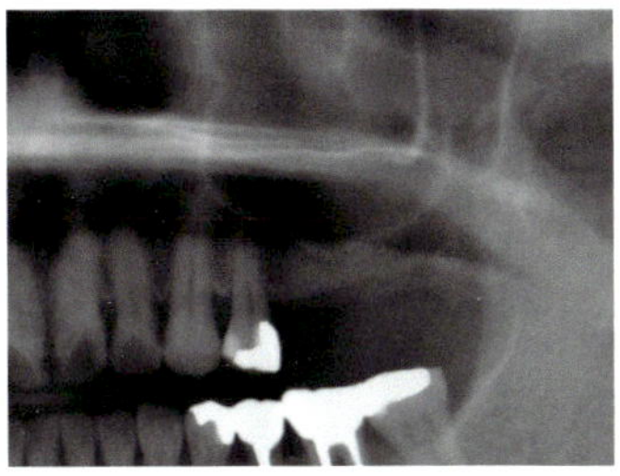

**Fig 4-10** Panoramic view after extraction of tooth 27.

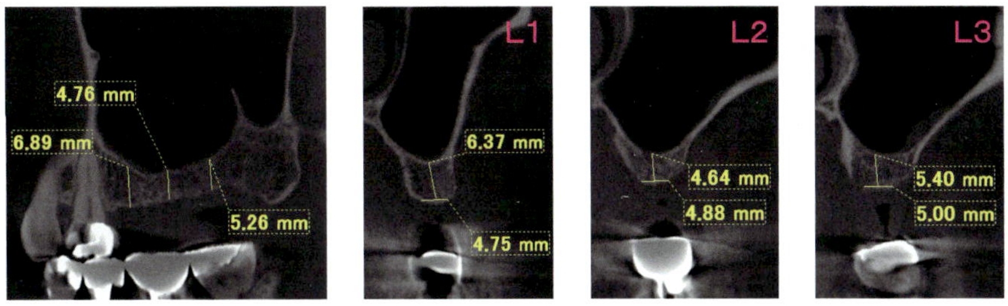


**Figs 4-11 to 4-14** CT images.

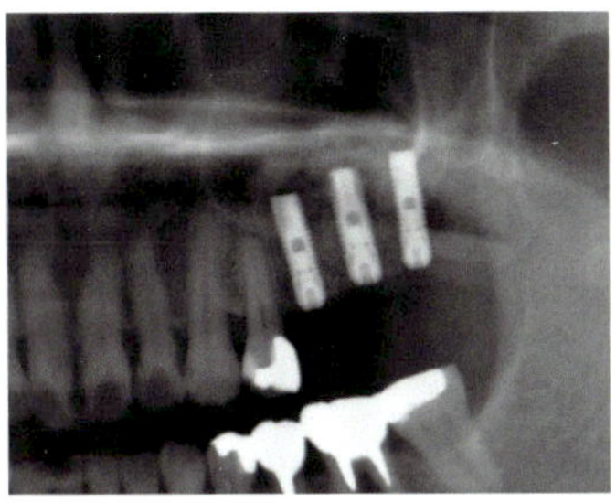

**Fig 4-15** Panoramic view immediately after surgery.

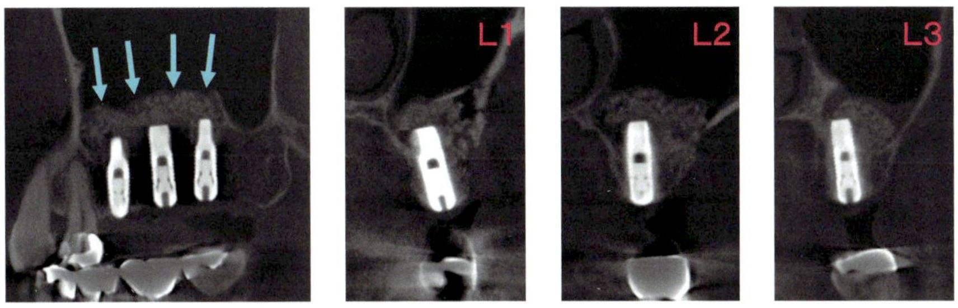


**Figs 4-16 to 4-19** CT images.

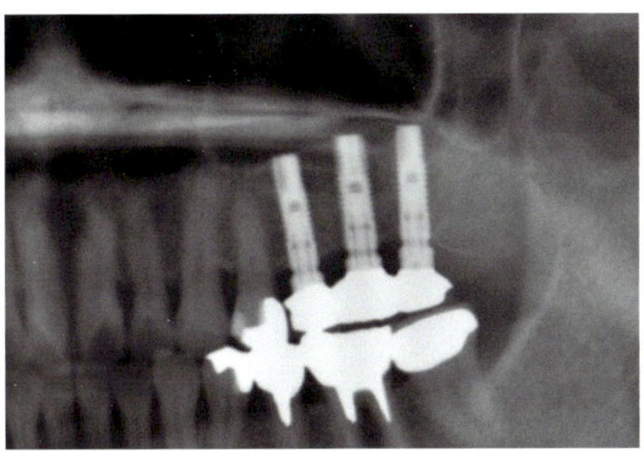

**Fig 4-20** Panoramic view 3 years after our surgery.

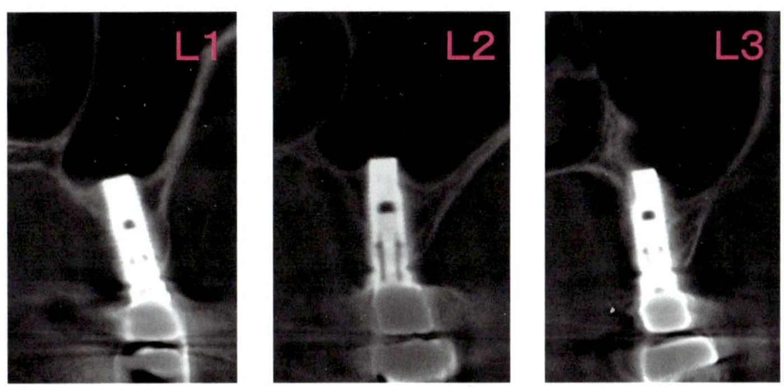


**Figs 4-21 to 4-23** CT images.

Shown next are the panoramic radiograph and CT images taken immediately after surgery (Figs 4-15 to 4-19). Good primary stability was attained, permitting the implant to be inserted simultaneously with sinus floor elevation.

Three implants were placed anterior to the septum, which was seen posteriorly in the maxillary sinus cavity, and 2 g of beta-tricalcium phosphate (β-TCP) was used to fill in the space (blue arrows on Fig 4-16). The buccolingual CT images clearly visualized the β-TCP granules around the implant apices (Figs 4-17 to 4-19). Due to a large mandibular arch, the implants were inserted at an angle to accept superstructures designed for occlusal cross-bite relationships.

A further postoperative panoramic radiograph and CT images taken 3 years after surgery are shown next (Figs 4-20 to 4-23). Although slight resorption is observed in the augmented area, the β-TCP granules have transformed into bone with a radiopacity level similar to that of cortical and cancellous bones.

## Check point 3: Mucous retention cyst

In this case, cysts were removed before sinus floor elevation to prevent cyst rupture during the elevation.

The patient had a long history of edentulism from tooth 14 to tooth 17, and was referred for implant treatment. The panoramic radiograph taken during the

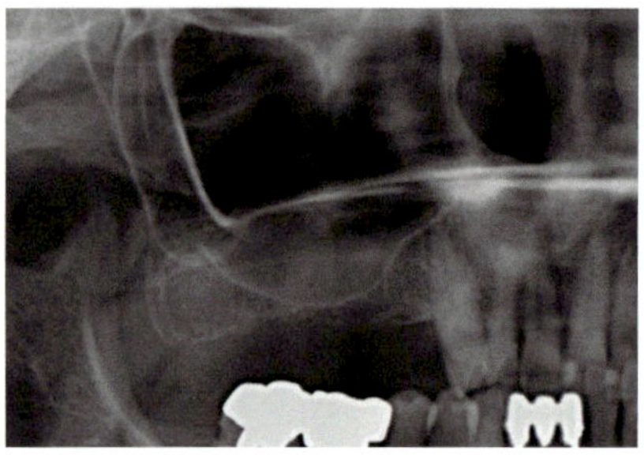

**Fig 4-24** Panoramic view before our surgery.

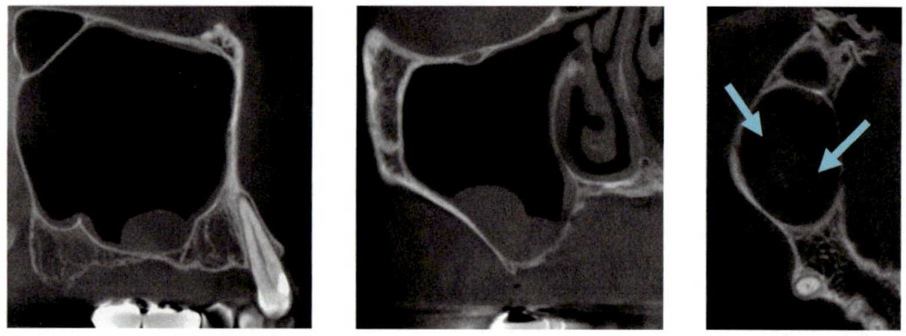

**Figs 4-25 to 4-27** CT images.

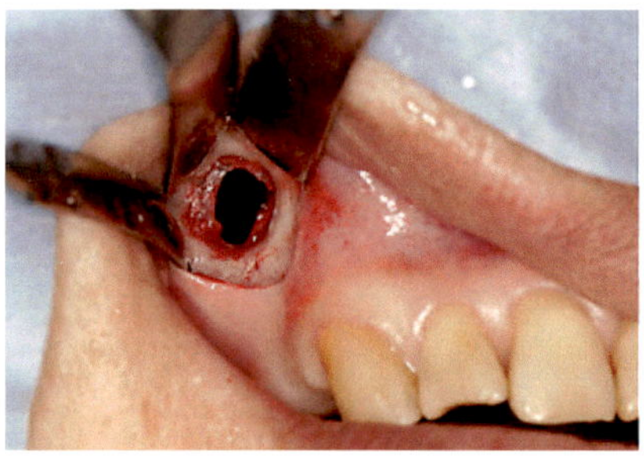

**Fig 4-28** Creating the osteotomy.

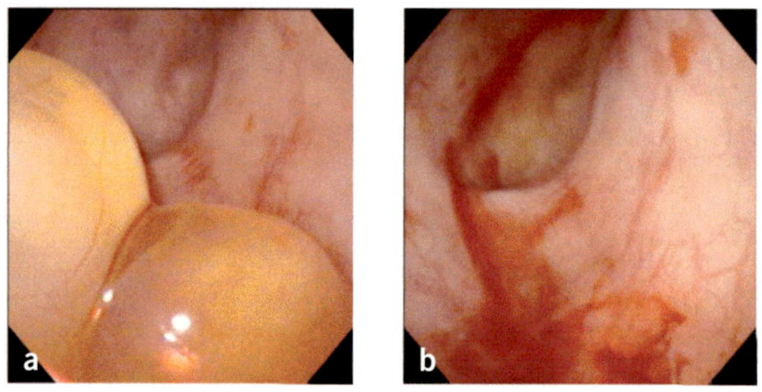


**Fig 4-29** (a and b) Fiberscope views before and after cyst removal.

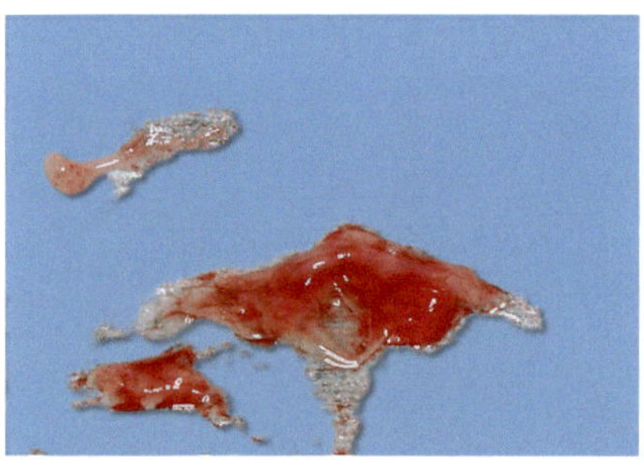

**Fig 4-30** Cyst removal with forceps.

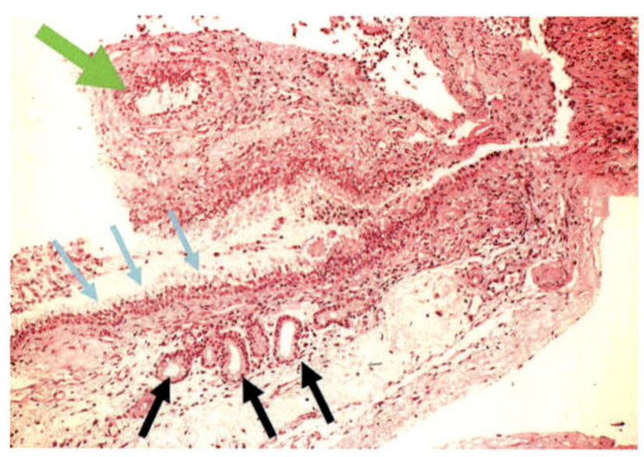

**Fig 4-31** Histopathological analysis of the cyst wall.

initial consultation indicated a dome-shaped radiopacity in the region extending from 15 to 17 (Fig 4-24). On CT imaging (Figs 4-25 to 4-27), a dome-shaped sessile radiopacity was found at two locations on the sinus floor (blue arrows on Fig 4-27), and they were determined to be mucous retention cysts.

Sinus floor elevation was necessary to increase the bone height for implant placement. Due to the risk of rupturing the cysts during dissection of the sinus membrane, cyst removal was performed prior to sinus floor elevation.

**! Key Point**

Employ a nasopharyngeal fiberscope for cyst removal.

**! Key Point**

Only a vertical incision was made to minimize the bleeding. Nasopharyngeal fiberscopy is useful in confirming the presence, and complete removal, of a cyst.

Following a vertical incision at region 14, an osteotomy of a diameter of about 8 mm was made over the canine fossa to create an access hole into the maxillary sinus cavity (Fig 4-28). A nasopharyngeal fiberscope inserted through the bone opening detected two cysts containing clear yellowish mucosal fluid (Fig 4-29a). The cysts could not be removed with the probe of the fiberscope, but were removed with nasopharyngeal forceps (Fig 4-30). Rupture of

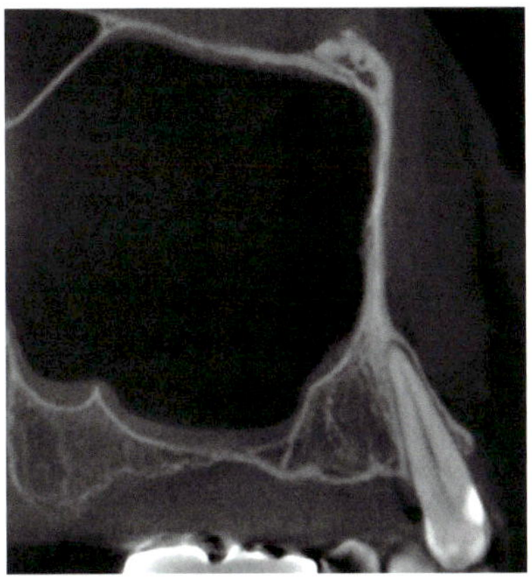

**Fig 4-32** Immediately after surgery.

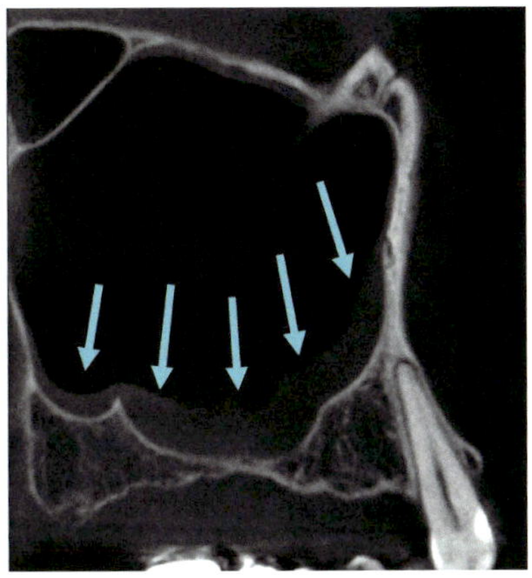

**Fig 4-33** One week after surgery.

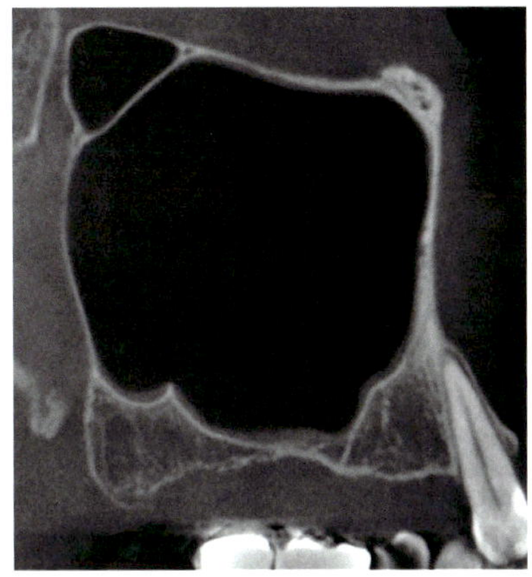

**Fig 4-34** Four months after surgery.

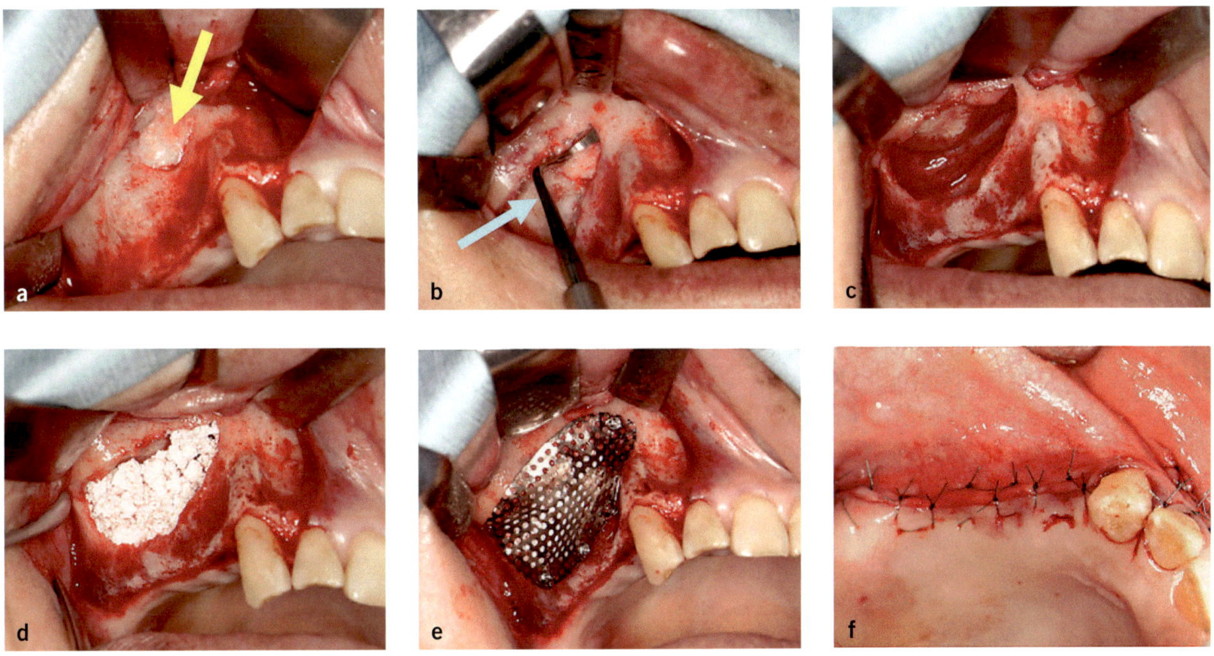

**Fig 4-35** (a to f) Intraoral views of the bone defect treatment.

the cysts was unavoidable as they were removed with their walls being grasped by the forceps. The lesion was checked again through the fiberscope to ensure complete cyst removal (Fig 4-29b), and the wound was then closed. The cyst wall was quite thin; histopathological analysis of the wall (Fig 4-31) revealed pseudostratified ciliated epithelium (blue arrows), mucus-producing cells (green arrows), and dilated ducts (black arrows).

Further sagittal images show postoperative follow-up immediately after surgery (Fig 4-32), 1 week later (Fig 4-33), and 4 months later (Fig 4-34). The CT image taken 1 week after removing the cyst demonstrated a temporary swelling of the maxillary sinus membrane (blue arrows on Fig 4-33). On the later CT image, membrane swelling was no longer observed and there was no sign of cyst recurrence.

**! Key Point**

Be aware of possible bone defects during cyst removal.

A bone defect was discovered on the maxillary sinus anterior wall where the access hole was created for cyst removal. A sharp dissection of the scar tissue was made at this region and a mucoperiosteal flap was reflected with extreme caution to prevent damage to the sinus membrane (yellow arrow on Fig 4-35a). After creating the lateral window, the sinus membrane was elevated using a small scalpel (KLS Martin; blue arrow on Fig 4-35b). The sinus membrane on the medial wall was also fully elevated and the empty space was filled with β-TCP (Fig 4-35d). A

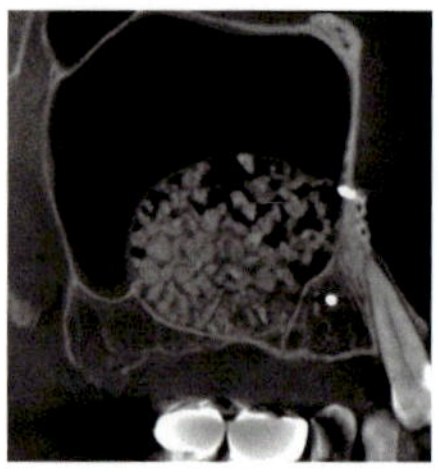

**Fig 4-36** Immediately after surgery.

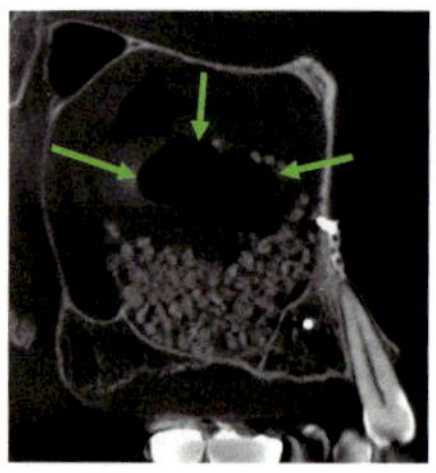

**Fig 4-37** One week after surgery.

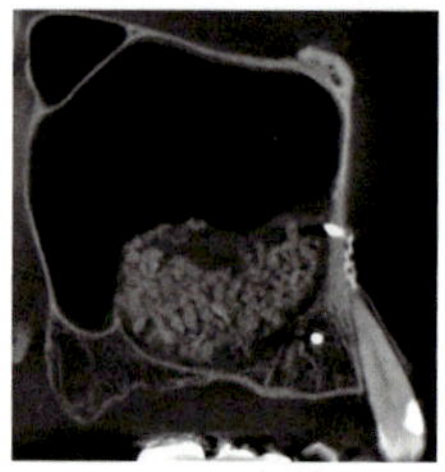

**Fig 4-38** Three months after surgery.

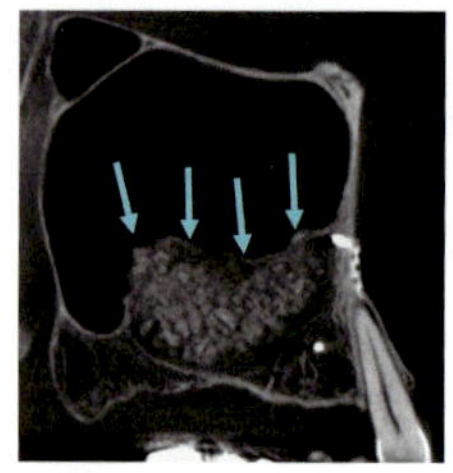

**Fig 4-39** Six months after surgery.

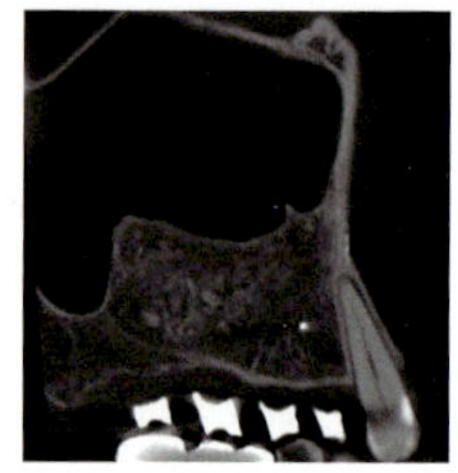

**Fig 4-40** One year after surgery.

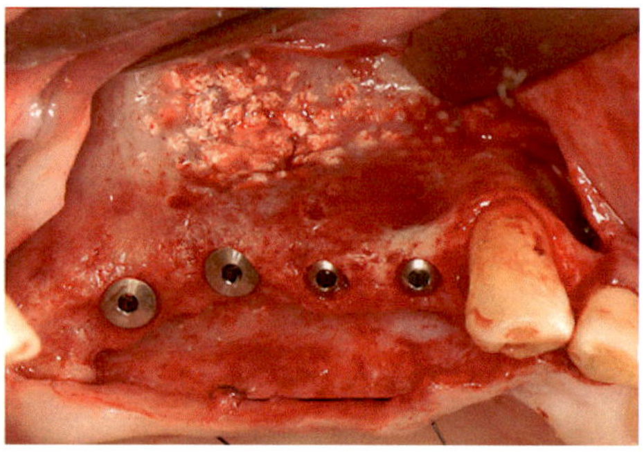

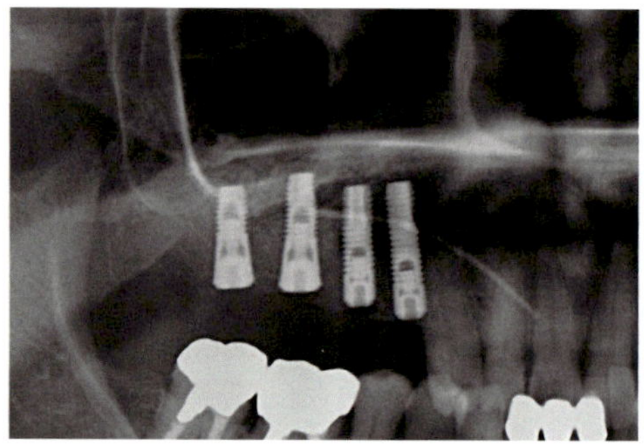

**Fig 4-41** (left) Intraoral view of the implants immediately after surgery.

**Fig 4-42** (right) Panoramic view of the implants immediately after surgery.

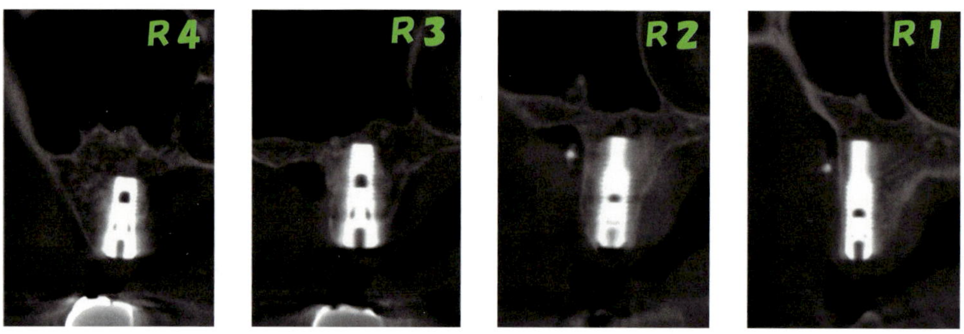


**Figs 4-43 to 4-46** Buccolingual images immediately after surgery.

titanium mesh plate was inserted over the lateral window and fixed in place with micro-screws (Pro-Seed, Japan; Fig 4-35e). The wound was then closed with sutures (Fig 4-35f).

CT images were taken again after the sinus floor elevation. Immediately after surgery, the radiopaque β-TCP granules, surrounded by air, were clearly visible directly beneath the elevated sinus membrane (Fig 4-36). After 1 week, postoperative swelling of the sinus membrane was observed and air was now trapped within the upper area of the cavity (green arrows on Fig 4-37. Three months following surgery, the membrane swelling had disappeared and the trapped air had been spontaneously resorbed (Fig 4-38). After 6 months, a thin radiopaque line was observed along the newly formed sinus floor (blue arrows on Fig 4-39), and the β-TCP granules in the marginal area were reduced in size. After 1 year, the radiopaque line along the newly formed sinus floor was more defined, whereas the cortical plate line of the original sinus floor was blurring (Fig 4-40). The β-TCP granules in the marginal area are seen to be further reduced in size. At the center of the figure, however, the remaining β-TCP granules are clearly seen. The clinical course after the lateral window technique was good with no sign of recurrence of the retention cysts.

One year after surgery, the titanium mesh was removed and four implants were inserted. All four implants attained good primary stability (Figs 4-41 and 4-42). Newly formed bone immediately beneath the titanium mesh incorporated some β-TCP granules, and its surface hardness was comparatively high (Fig 4-41). Buccolingual CT images taken immediately after implant placement confirmed that all implants were located within the bone (Figs 4-43 to 4-46).

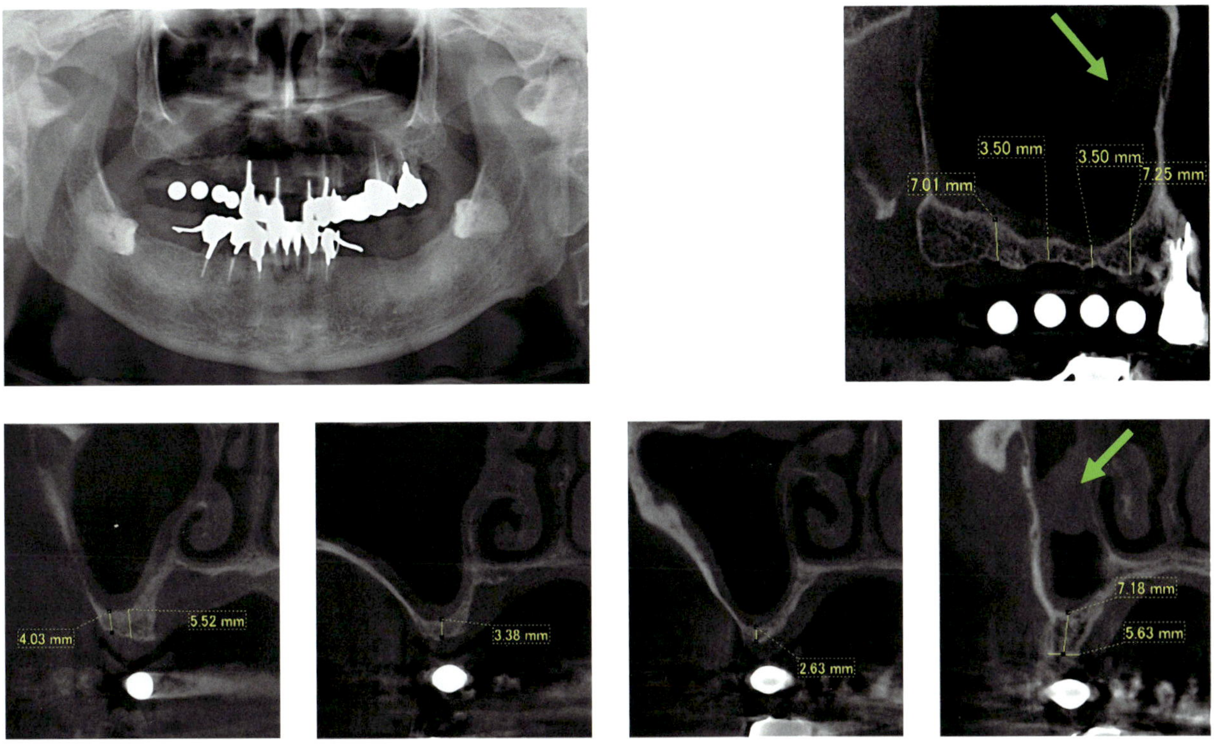


**Figs 4-47 to 4-52** Panoramic view and CT images at the diagnosis.

## Check point 4: Maxillary sinusitis

This patient with a long history of edentulism from tooth 14 to tooth 18 was referred for implant treatment (Figs 4-47 to 4-52). The patient had a history of chronic maxillary sinusitis and was being treated with antibiotics, including macrolide.

CT revealed slight thickening of the sinus membrane and a retention-cyst–like radiopacity in the upper area (green arrows on Figs 4-48 and 4-52). The ENT doctor's opinion was that the membrane thickening had been improved and would not negatively impact sinus floor elevation surgery. Based on the findings that the retention-cyst–like radiopacity was in the upper area and that the membrane swelling was uniform with no edema, it was determined that the sinus floor elevation could be performed safely.

On the day set for the sinus floor elevation, the patient mentioned a mild cold he had had 5 days earlier. He said that he had already recovered from the cold and had no symptoms such as sore throat, fever or sense of fatigue. However, considering the fact that only 5 days had passed since he had the respiratory infection, and that he had a history of chronic maxillary sinusitis, we decided to take a CT scan before the surgery.

**! Key Point**

Be cautious about upper airway respiratory infections. Don't take maxillary sinusitis lightly!

The sinus membrane presented significant swelling (yellow arrows on Figs 4-53 and 4-54) and the sur-

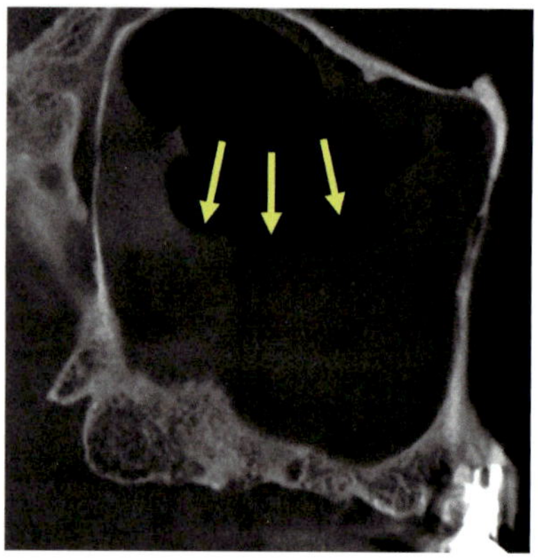
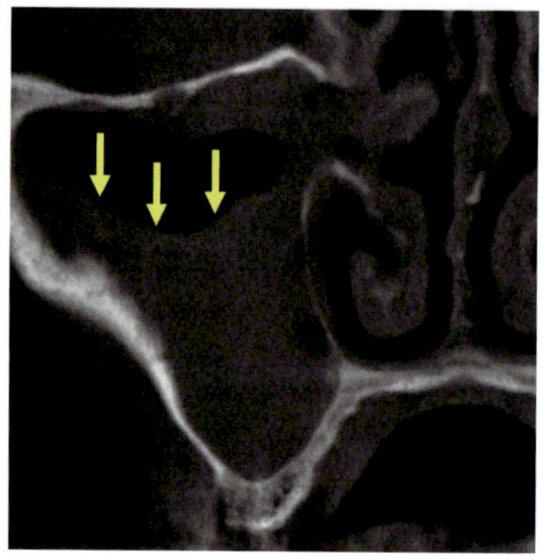

**Figs 4-53 and 4-54** CT scans showing significant swelling of the sinus membrane.

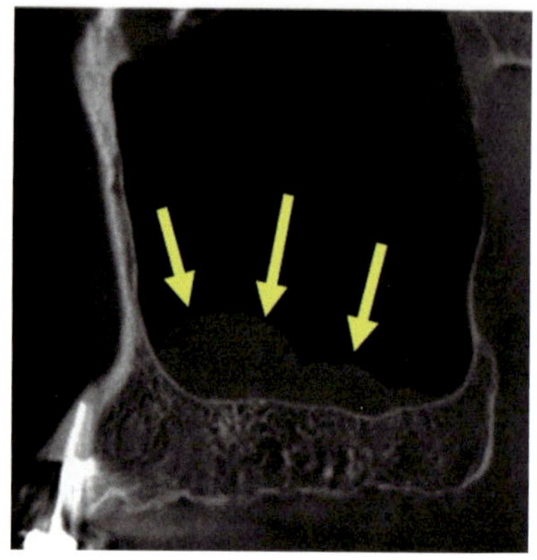

**Fig 4-55** CT image prior to surgery.

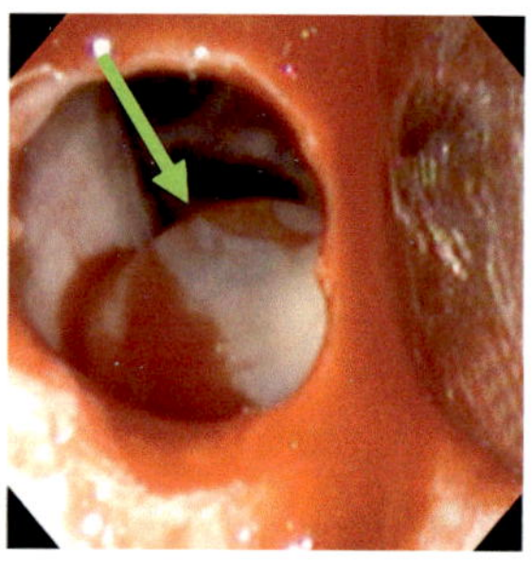
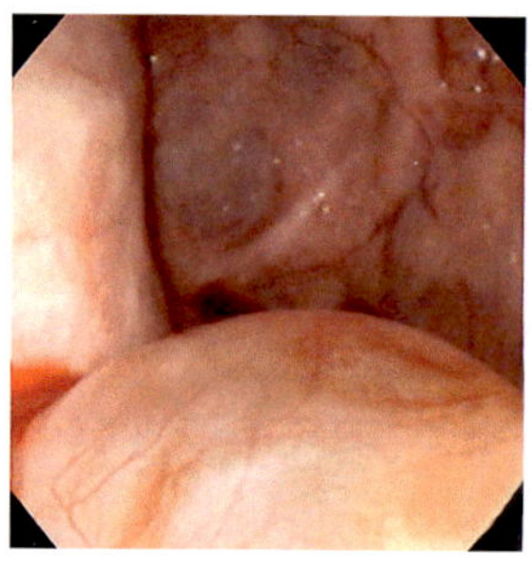

**Figs 4-56 and 4-57** (left and middle) Intraoral views revealing a whitish mass.

**Fig 4-58** (right) Removal of the mass.

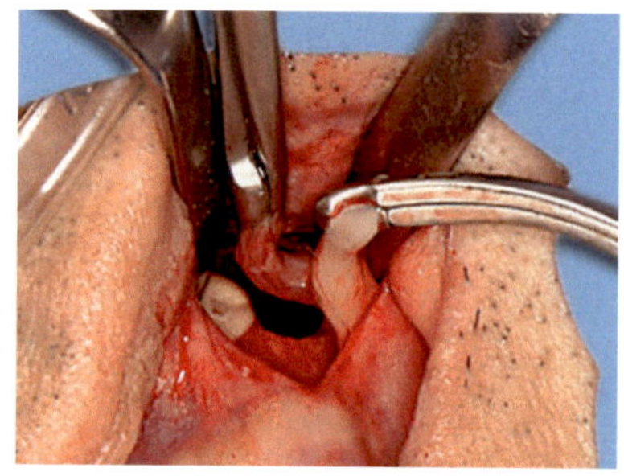

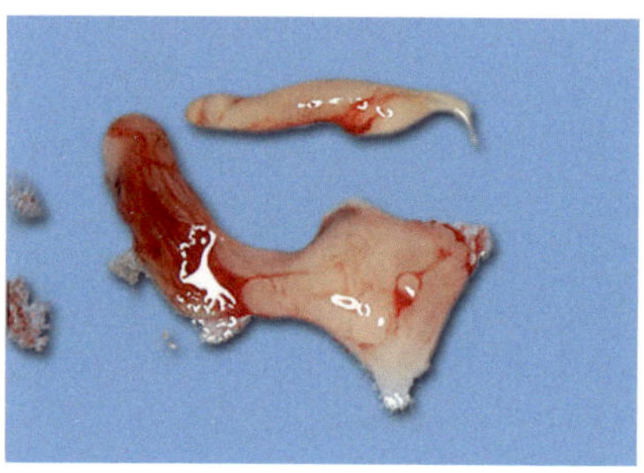
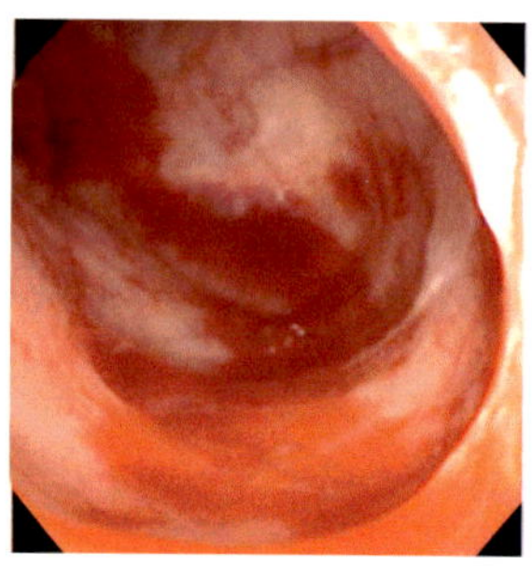

**Figs 4-59 and 4-60** Fluid inside the cyst was viscous and had a milky color.

gery was postponed, while informing the patient of the risks associated with elevating the affected sinus membrane. If these CT scans had not been done, there is no doubt that sinus floor elevation would have been performed as scheduled and resulted in problems.

> **! Key Point**
>
> Preoperative CT examination is usually performed 1 month before surgery. It should be noted, however, that the condition of the maxillary sinus membrane can change quickly.

## Check point 5: CT cannot identify the fluid inside a retention cyst

There is a school of thought that the fluid contained in cysts can be removed during a sinus floor elevation procedure, so there is no need for prior removal. However, even if retention-cyst–like radiopacity is shown on a CT image, it is impossible to know whether the fluid is non-infectious.

This patient was referred for preoperative CT examination prior to implant placement. The first CT image revealed a dome-shaped radiopacity in the sinus cavity (yellow arrows on Fig 4-55). Based on the judgment that it was a mucous retention cyst, surgery for cyst removal was performed by creating an access hole at the canine fossa. Through a

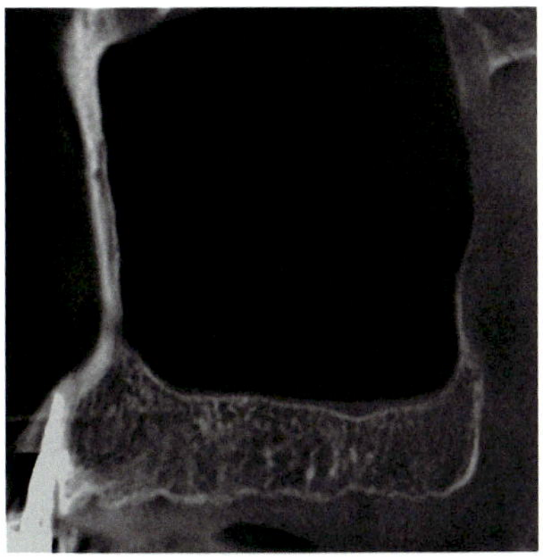

Fig 4-61 (left) Immediately after surgery for cyst removal.

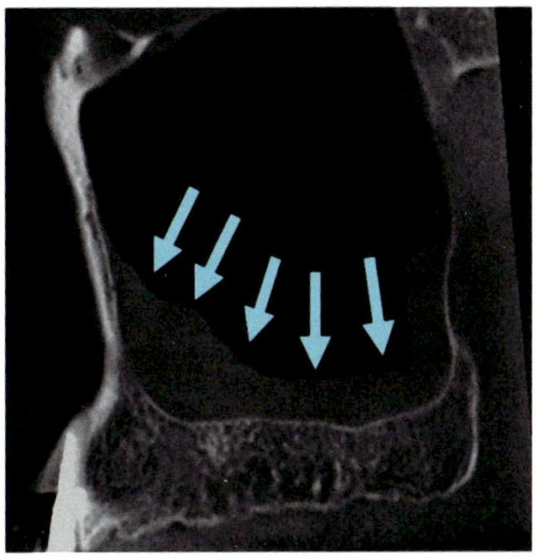

Fig 4-62 (right) One week after surgery for cyst removal.

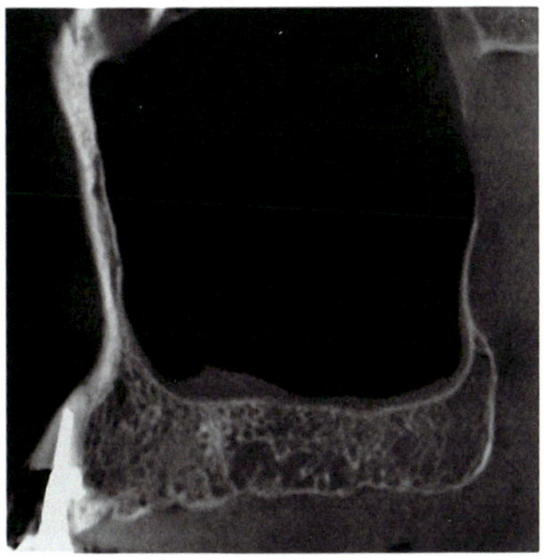

Fig 4-63 (left) One month after surgery for cyst removal.

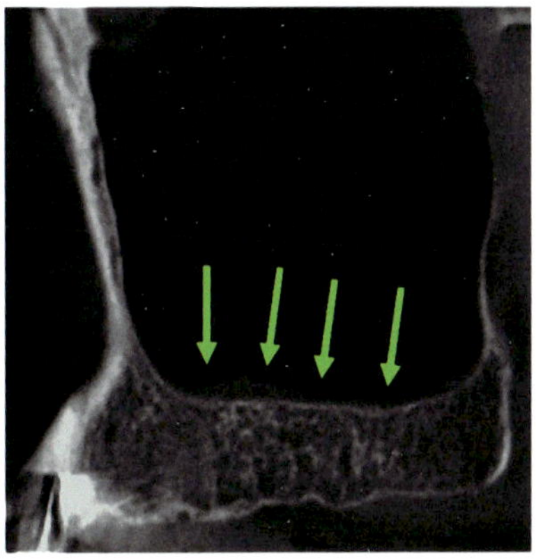

Fig 4-64 (right) Four months after surgery for cyst removal.

fiberscope, a whitish mass was found inside the sinus cavity and the fluid inside the mass appeared translucent (Figs 4-56 and 4-57). However, the fluid inside the removed cyst was actually viscous and possessed a milky color, indicative of microbial infection (Figs 4-58 and 4-59).

This demonstrates that, while CT scans are valuable in detecting mucous retention cysts, they are not capable of evaluating the fluid inside the cyst. The author believes that any mucous retention cyst should be removed before a sinus floor elevation procedure to avoid the risk of postoperative infection.

The CT image taken immediately after surgery indicates complete removal of the cyst (Fig 4-61). The maxillary sinus membrane at 1 week shows swelling induced by mechanical stimulation during cyst removal (blue arrows on Fig 4-62). The membrane swelling improved, as evidenced by the 1-month postoperative CT image (Fig 4-63) and was almost absent on the 4-month CT image (green arrows on Fig 4-64).

**! Key Point**

In cases of retention cyst removal, the author makes it a rule to allow the sinus membrane to heal and stabilize for 4 months prior to undertaking sinus floor elevation. However, the possibility of cyst recurrence cannot be ruled out, so follow-up by CT examination is essential.

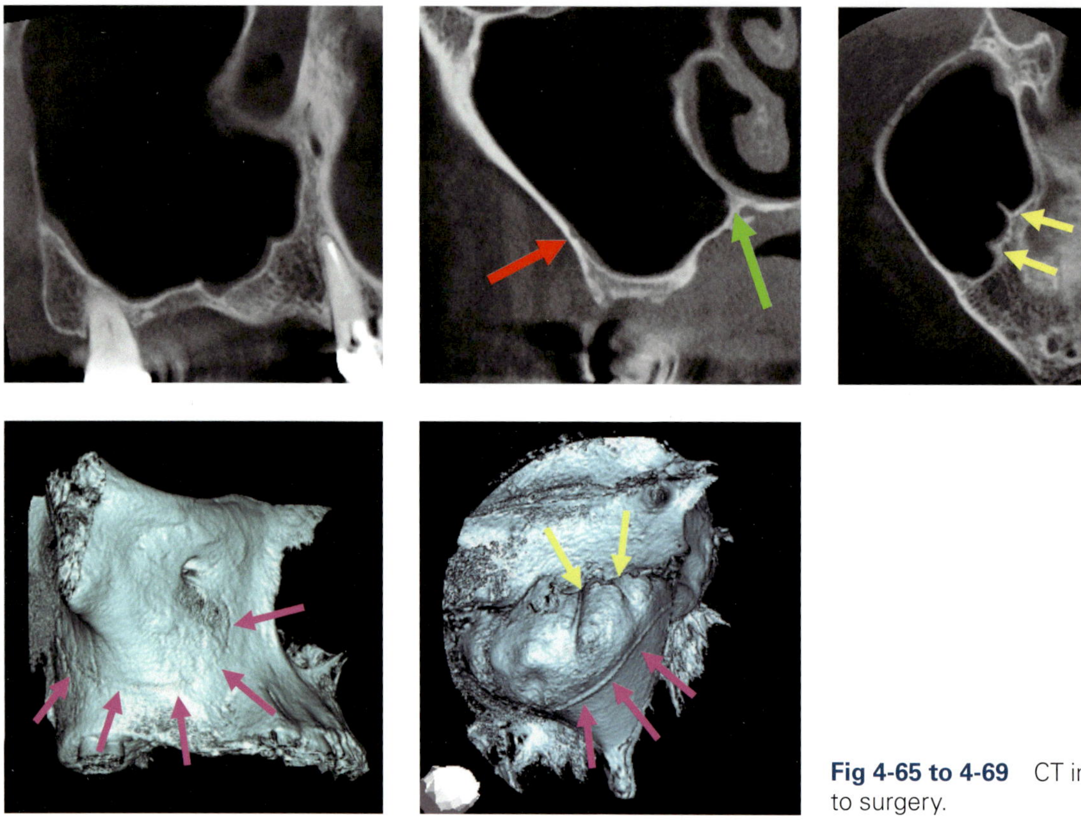

**Fig 4-65 to 4-69** CT images prior to surgery.

## 4.2 The intraoperative stage

### Introduction

Prior to commencing sinus floor elevation by the lateral window technique, it is crucial to be fully aware where the superior alveolar artery runs along the anterior wall of the maxillary sinus. When the superior alveolar artery passes transversely over the lateral window and no bone is present medial to the artery, the artery can be dissected from the bone surface to elevate the lateral window. In contrast, if bone is present medial to the artery, it is impossible to dissect the artery from the bone surface and the lateral window cannot be elevated, necessitating alternative surgical procedures.

> **! Key Point**
>
> Buccolingual CT scans are indispensable, not only for determining the arterial route but also the presence or absence of bone medial to the artery.

### Procedure when no bone is present medial to superior alveolar artery

> **! Key Point**
>
> If there is no bone medial to the artery (red arrow on Fig 4-66), the artery may be dissected from the bone surface.

This patient presented with loss of teeth 15 to 17, and required sinus floor elevation (Fig 4-65). Preoperative CT scans revealed downward and inward growth of the maxillary sinus (green arrow on Fig 4-66) and the presence of the septa (yellow arrows on Figs 4-67 and 4-69). The superior alveolar artery passed transversely along the anterior wall of the maxillary sinus (pink arrows on Figs 4-68 and 4-69), the route of which coincided with the site of the proposed lateral window. The buccolingual CT image showed no bone medial to the artery (red arrow on Fig 4-66), which indicated that the artery was in direct contact with the sinus membrane.

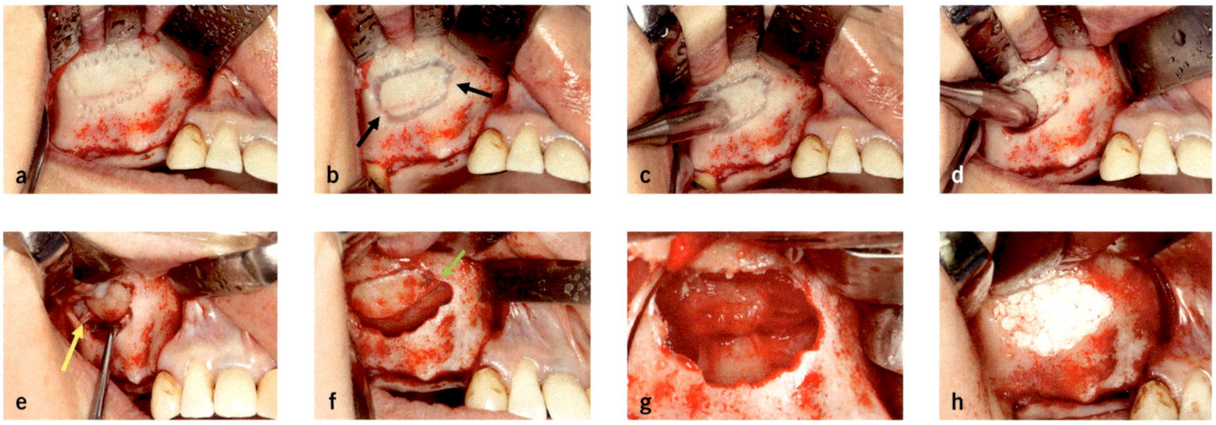


**Figs 4-70a–h** Intraoral views during the surgery.

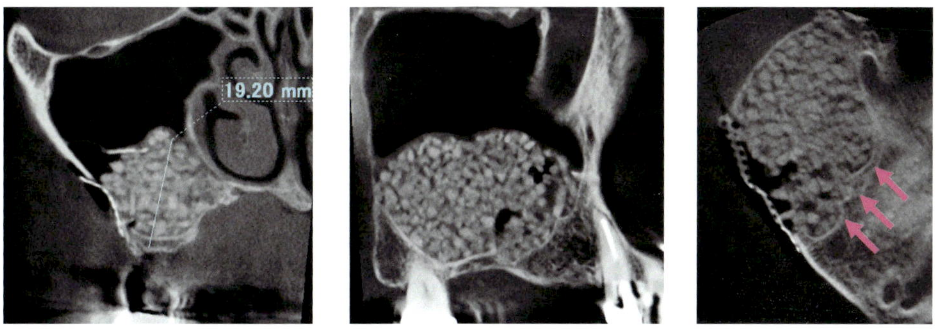


**Figs 4-71 to 4-73** Postoperative CT images.

### ! Key Point

At locations where the superior alveolar artery is present, care must be taken during drilling to avoid injury of the artery (Fig 4-70a).

In this patient, the superior alveolar artery was found immediately beneath the bone surface and the route coincided with the osteotomy line where the lateral window was to be created. Using a diamond round bur, dot-like drillings were made. At locations where the superior alveolar artery was passing, drillings were made in such a way as to avoid interference with the artery (Fig 4-70a). To avoid damage to the artery, the thin bone plate was left intact around the artery (black arrows on Fig 4-70b). The lateral window was fractured inward by gentle tapping (Fig 4-70c).

By gently pressing the lateral window medially, the sinus membrane and the artery around the lateral window were dissected spontaneously (Fig 4-70d). Should any damage occur to the artery, hemostasis by pressing the blood vessel is difficult. The use of an electrosurgical knife would be useful. Due to adhesion of the superior alveolar artery and sinus membrane, the artery was dissected together with the membrane using a small scalpel (yellow arrow on Fig 4-70e).

The artery anterior to the lateral window was also separated from the bone surface (green arrow on Fig 4-70f). When no bone is present medial to the superior alveolar artery on the buccolingual CT image, as was the case for this patient, the artery can be dissected together with the maxillary sinus membrane.

Successful dissection of the superior alveolar artery enabled sufficient reflection of the sinus membrane from the septa of the medial wall (Fig 4-70g). A sufficient amount of β-TCP granules was placed directly beneath the elevated sinus membrane (Fig 4-70h).

Postoperative CT images show the situation immediately after the sinus floor elevation (Figs 4-71 to 4-73). Titanium mesh was fixed with micro-screws over the lateral window. A sufficient amount of grafting material was placed into the created space and radiopaque β-TCP granules can be seen peripheral to the septa (pink arrows on Fig 4-73).

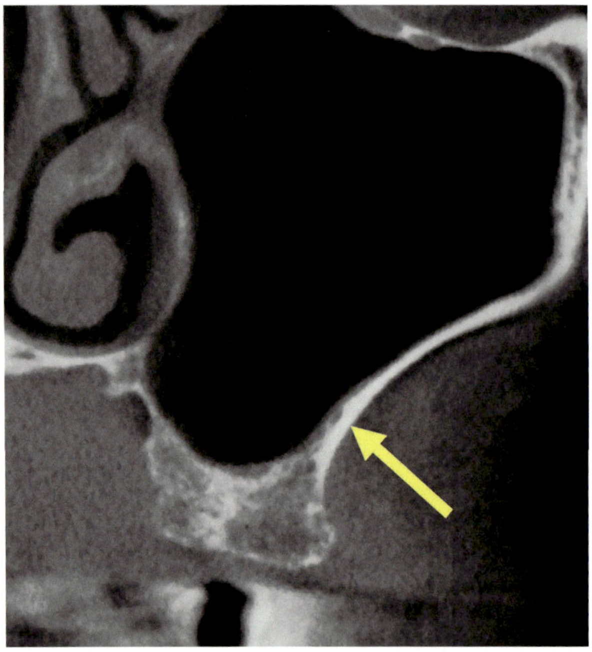

**Fig 4-74** Preoperative CT scan shows a thin bone plate medial to the superior alveolar artery.

## Procedure when bone is present medial to superior alveolar artery

> **! Key Point**
>
> Bone plate medial to the superior alveolar artery makes it challenging to separate the artery from the bone surface, resulting in difficulties with lateral window elevation.

In this patient, a preoperative buccolingual CT image revealed a thin bone plate medial to the superior alveolar artery (yellow arrow on Fig 4-74). When the bone plate is present medial to the anterior superior alveolar artery, such as in this case, it is difficult to separate the artery from the bone surface, which makes lateral window elevation difficult.

> **! Key Point**
>
> Ligate and cut the superior alveolar artery after extending it as far as possible.

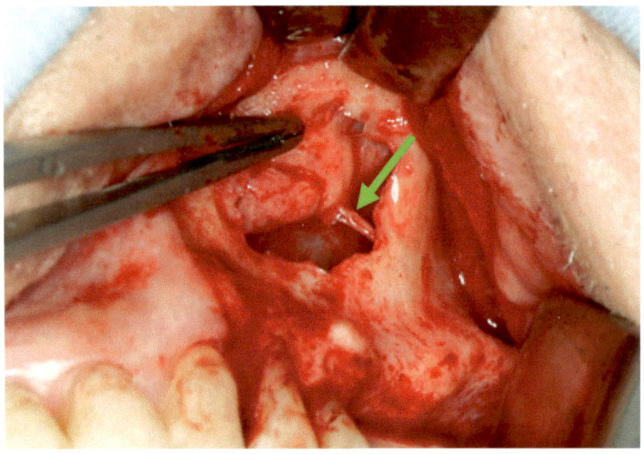

**Fig 4-75** Intraoral view of the superior alveolar artery.

The superior alveolar artery was extended as far as possible (green arrow on Fig 4-75), and then ligated and cut so as to facilitate lateral window elevation. A postoperative CT image shows a sufficient amount of β-TCP granules in the created space (Fig 4-76). This case demonstrates that preoperative buccolingual CT scans are not only useful to find the route of the superior alveolar artery but also to determine the presence or absence of bone medial to the artery.

## Complicated maxillary sinus morphology (septum)

The morphology of the maxillary sinus floor differs from person to person, with some possessing sinus septa. Panoramic radiography cannot provide morphological information on the septum, so examination by CT scanning is indispensable.

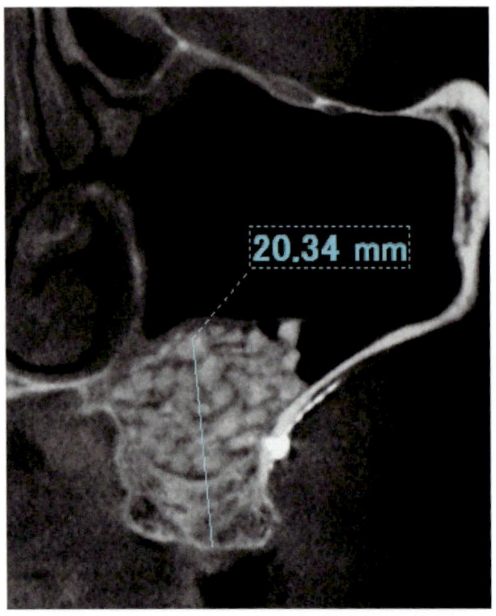


**Fig 4-76** Postoperative CT scan of the β-TCP granules in the created space.

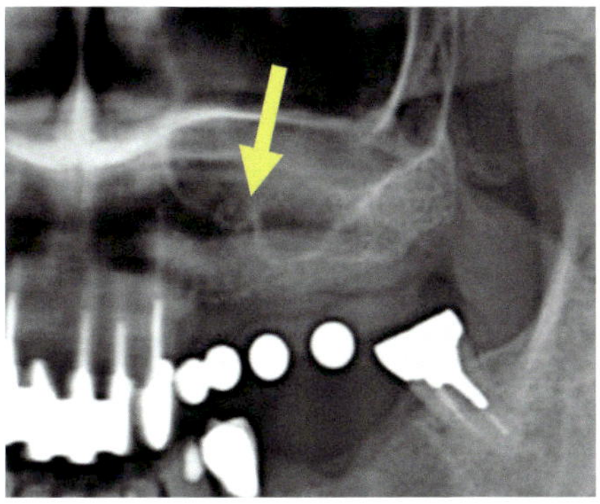

Fig 4-77 Preoperative panoramic view.

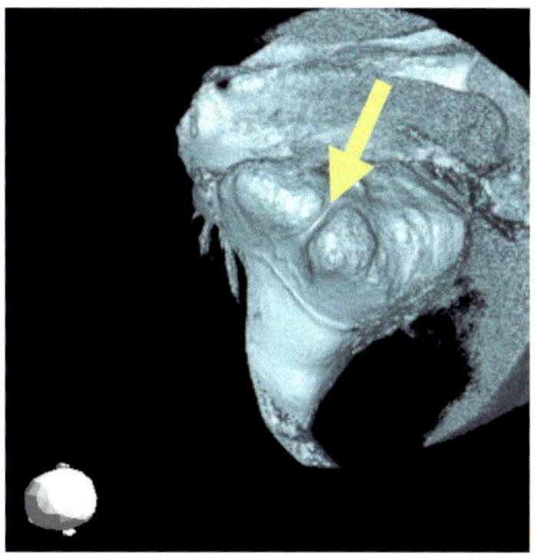

Fig 4-78 Preoperative volume rendering image.

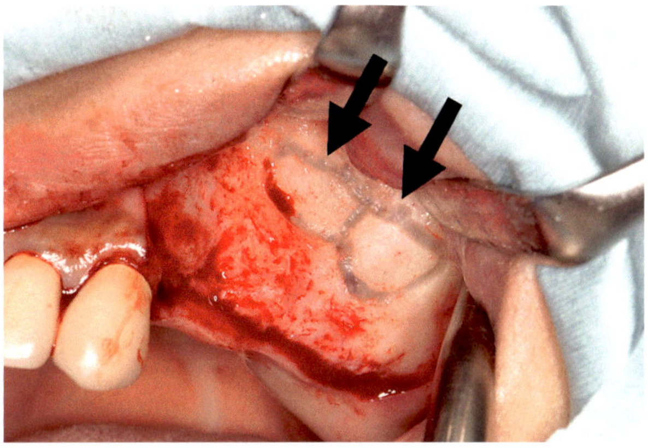

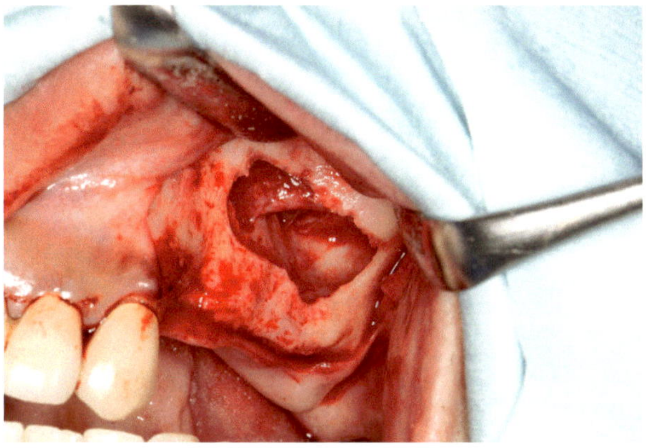

**Figs 4-79 and 4-80** Intraoperative intraoral views.

> **! Key Point**
>
> When a sinus septum is present, dissecting the sinus membrane in one direction by crossing the septum carries the risk of membrane perforation. Volume rendering CT images are useful for septum examination.

## Procedure when a septum is present

This patient was referred for implant placement involving sinus floor elevation to replace missing teeth 24 to 27. Placement of four implants was deemed necessary. Owing to the presence of a sinus septum between L2 and L3, sinus floor elevation by avoiding the septum was considered difficult (Fig 4-77). A volume rendering CT image indicated the presence of the septum in the buccolingual direction (yellow arrow on Fig 4-78) and the sinus floor had a concave appearance behind the septum. It was considered risky to dissect the sinus membrane by crossing the septum through the lateral window created in the front of the septum.

In this patient, two lateral windows were created to dissect the sinus membrane over the sinus septum from both the mesial and distal sides. The membrane on the crest of the septum was eventually dissected, thus avoiding membrane perforation (Figs 4-79 and 4-80).

> **! Key Point**
>
> Create two lateral windows.

## Procedure when there are two septa

This patient with loss of teeth 14 to 17 was treated using sinus floor elevation. A preoperative panoramic radiograph could not provide clear information on the morphology of the maxillary sinus (Fig 4-81). In contrast, the horizontal CT image revealed the presence of two large septa (Figs 4-82 to 4-84). The anterior septum ran obliquely inside the sinus cavity (green arrows on Figs 4-83 and 4-84), and the sinus membrane on the septum presented some thickening (yellow arrows on Fig 4-83). In addition, observing the maxillary sinus from above on the volume rendering image provided a complete image of the sinus floor morphology (Fig 4-85). Creation of two lateral windows was considered necessary for sinus membrane elevation in this patient.

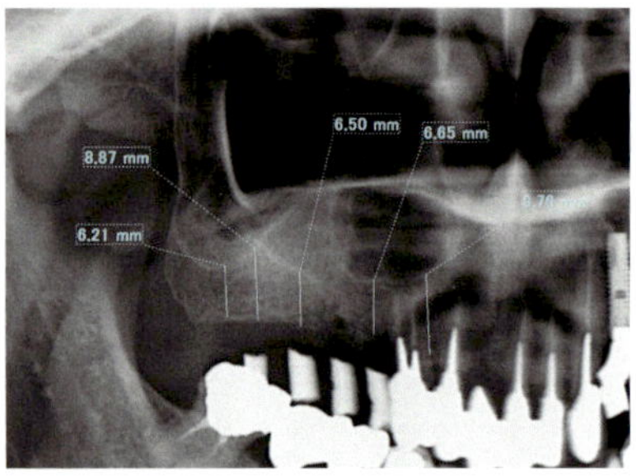


**Fig 4-81** Preoperative panoramic view.

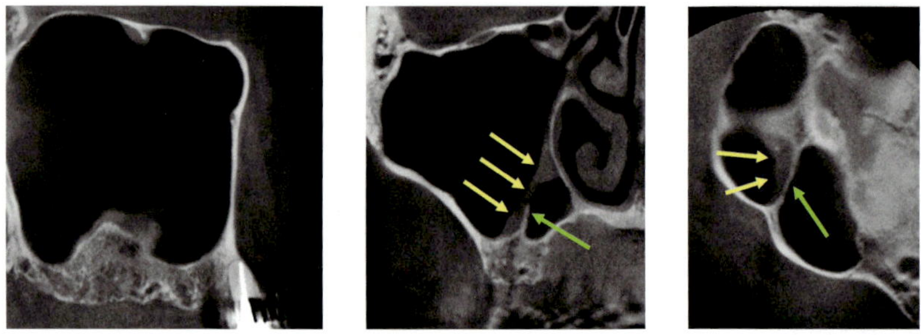

**Figs 4-82 to 4-84** Preoperative CT images showing two large septa.

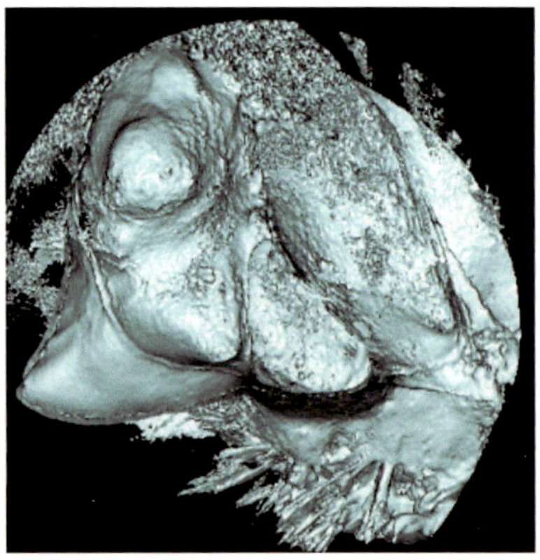

**Fig 4-85** Volume rendering image.

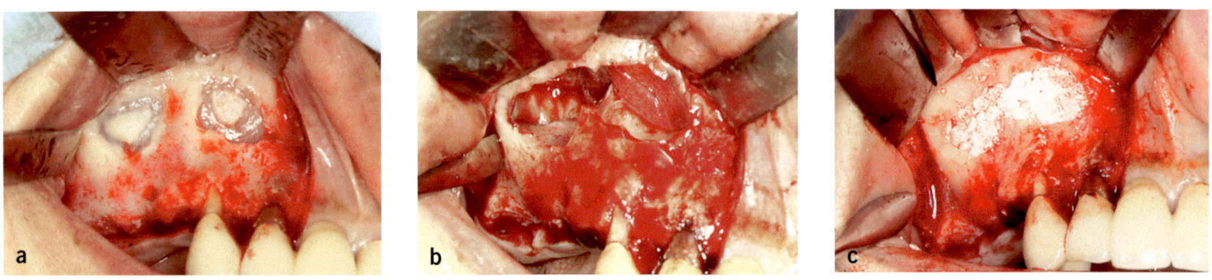


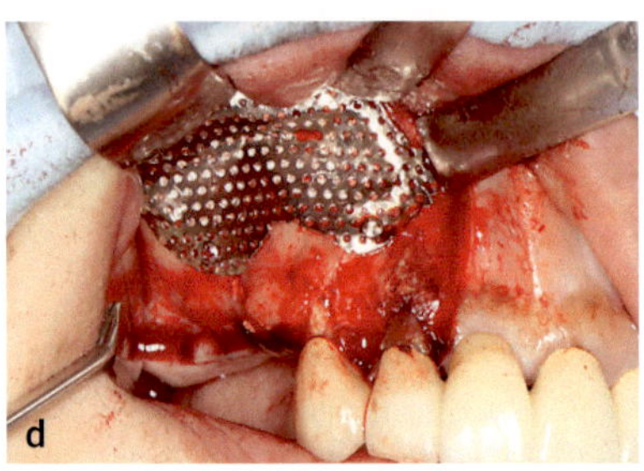


**Fig 4-86** (a to d) Intraoperative intraoral views.

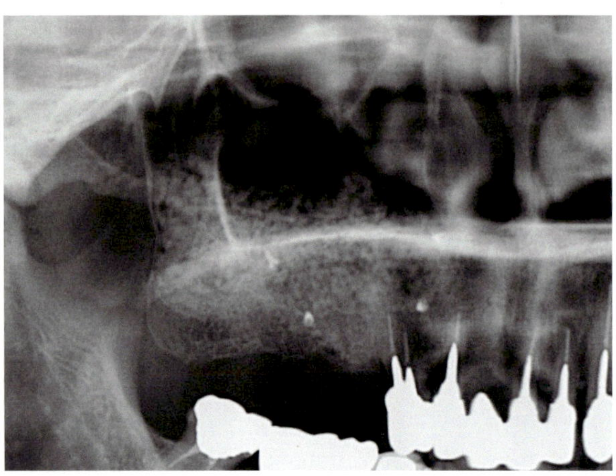

**Fig 4-87** Panoramic view immediately after surgery.

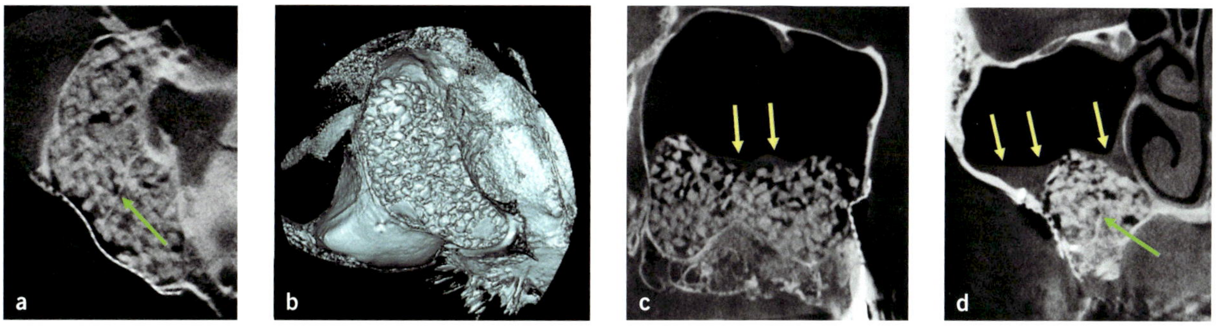


**Fig 4-88** (a to d) CT images immediately after surgery.

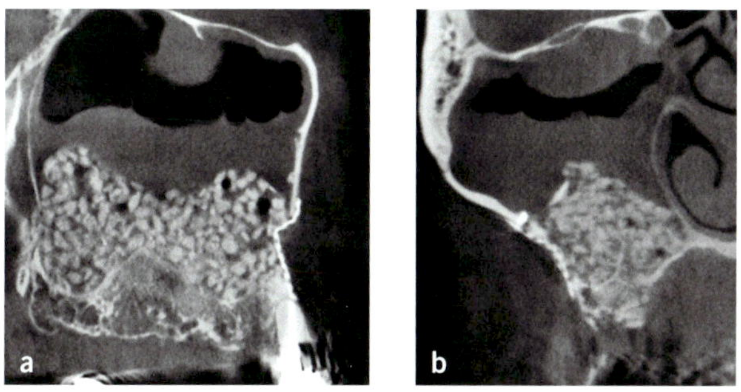


**Fig 4-89** (a and b) CT images 1 week after surgery.

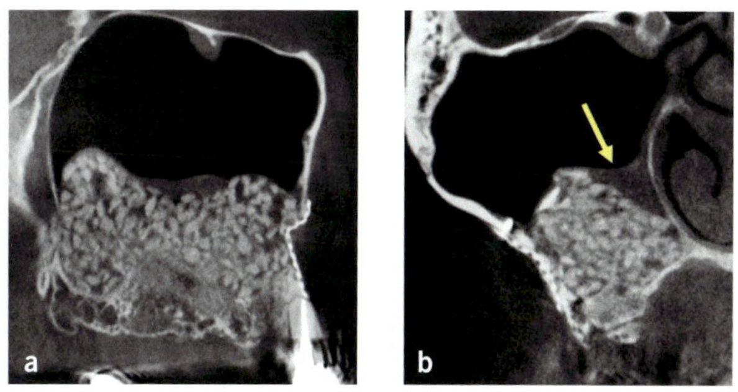


**Fig 4-90** (a and b) CT images 1 month after surgery.

A total of two lateral windows were created at the anterior and posterior sides of the canine, and the sinus membrane was elevated (Figs 4-86a and 4-86b). After placement of β-TCP granules, a titanium mesh was secured over the lateral window and affixed with micro-screws (Figs 4-86c and 4-86d).

> **! Key Point**
>
> Create one lateral window at the anterior side and the other at the posterior side of the canine.

Shown next are a panoramic radiograph and CT images taken immediately following surgery (Fig 4-87 and 4-88). A sufficient amount of β-TCP granules was placed in the created space and the thickened sinus membrane was elevated (yellow arrows on Figs 4-88c and d). Densely packed β-TCP granules were observed around the septa (green arrow on Fig 4-88d).

CT imaging 1 week later shows apparent swelling of the maxillary sinus membrane (Fig 4-89). One month after surgery, further CT images (Fig 4-90) show that the swelling had disappeared but the membrane thickening, which was observed before surgery, still partly remained (Fig 4-90a and yellow arrow on 4-90b).

## Procedure when maxillary sinus anterior wall is thick

External protrusion of the zygomaticoalveolar crest (ZAC) makes the creation of the lateral window difficult. Preoperative CT evaluation of the ZAC is essential. It should also be noted that osteotomy is more difficult when the anterior wall of the maxillary sinus is thicker.

This patient was referred for implant placements at positions 16 and 17. The planned implant sites presented inadequate bone height and required a sinus floor elevation by the lateral window technique (Fig 4-91). Owing to the presence of the ZAC, the anterior wall of the sinus was thick (red arrows on Figs 4-92 to 4-94).

> **! Key Point**
>
> Creation of a lateral window at the ZAC is difficult owing to the thickness of the sinus anterior wall, and poor visibility.

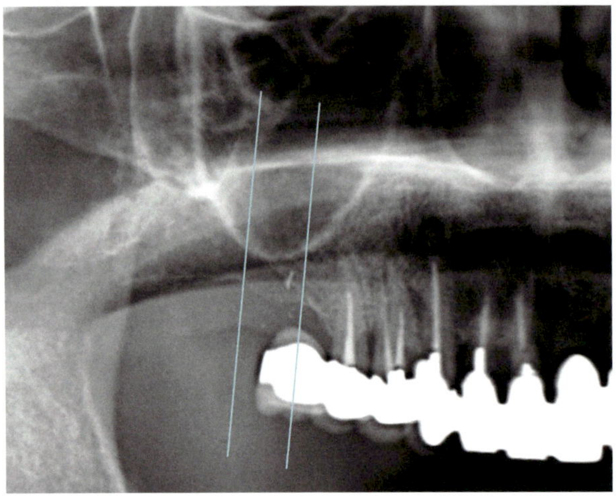

Fig 4-91 Panoramic view before our surgery.

> **! Key Point**
>
> Reduce the bone thickness beforehand if it is excessively thick. Trimming with a diamond round bur of a larger size is useful in reducing the thickness and making the lateral window creation easier.

Adequate vertical incision is required to ensure direct vision of the operative field (Figs 4-95a and b), and a skilled assistant is essential to securely reflect and hold the mucoperiosteal flap (Fig 4-95b and black ar-

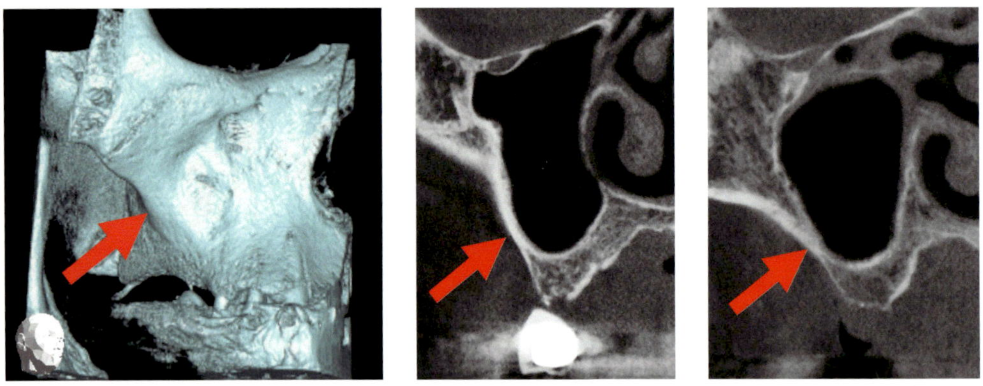

Figs 4-92 to 4-94 CT images before surgery.

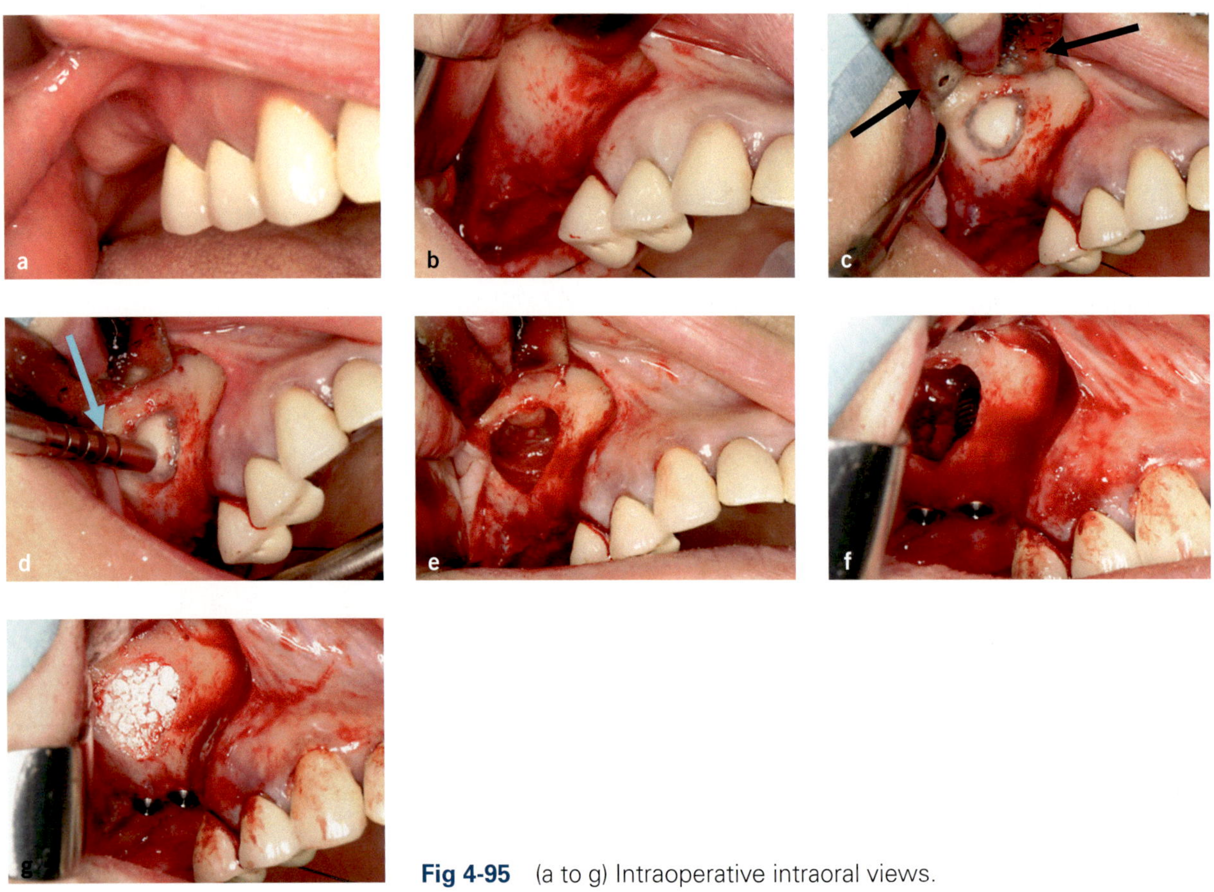

Fig 4-95 (a to g) Intraoperative intraoral views.

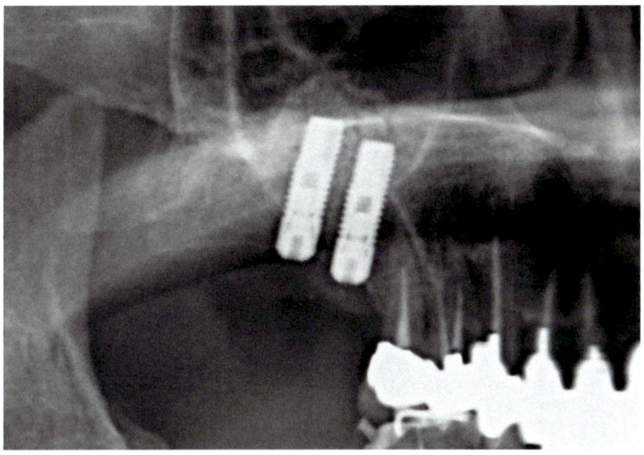

Fig 4-96 Postoperative panoramic view of the two implants.

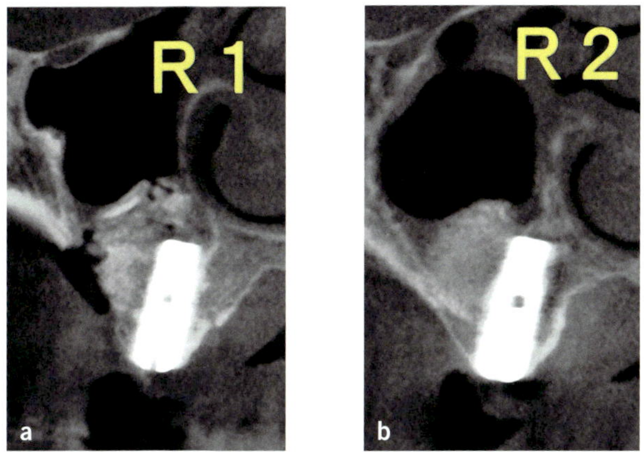


Fig 4-97 (a and b) CT images immediately after the surgery.

rows on Fig 4-95c). If the bone of the sinus anterior wall is too thick, trimming with a diamond round bur of a larger size is useful in reducing the thickness and making the lateral window creation easier. Fracture the lateral window by gently tapping with an instrument such as an osteotome (blue arrow on Fig 4-95d), then gently push the lateral window medially and dissect the sinus membrane around the lateral window.

Two implants were inserted after elevating the sinus membrane (Figs 4-95e and f). After confirming the good primary stability of the implants, β-TCP granules were placed around the implants and the wound was closed (Figs 4-95g and 4-96).

In cases where primary stability cannot be attained, the author believes it is safer to remove the implant and allow the augmented area to heal (to be described in a later section).

Images are shown of the postoperative follow-up, immediately after surgery, and at 6 months, 1 year and 2 years (Figs 4-97 to 4-100). R1 and R2 achieved osseointegration. Two years after the surgery, the region where β-TCP granules were placed showed radiopacities that indicated formation of cortical- and cancellous-like bones (blue arrows on Figs 4-100).

## Morphology of bone inside the sinus cavity

Sinus floor elevation is a form of bone augmentation employed to facilitate placement of an implant of adequate length. Insufficient dissection or elevation of the sinus membrane will make implant placement impossible.

When a maxillary posterior implant is placed from the alveolar crest in an axial direction toward the func-

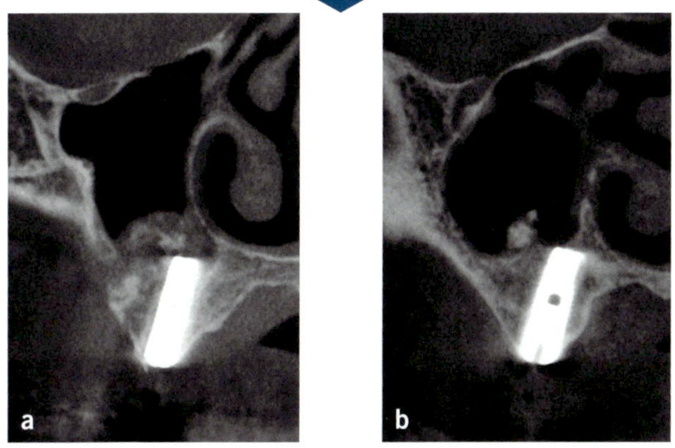


Fig 4-98 (a and b) Postoperative CT images at 6 months.

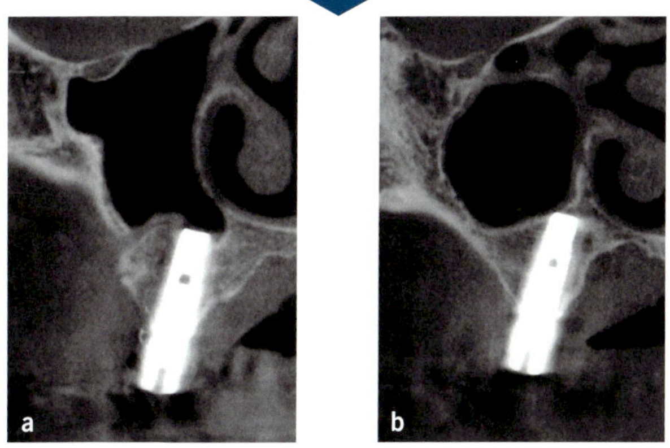


Fig 4-99 (a and b) Postoperative CT images at 1 year.

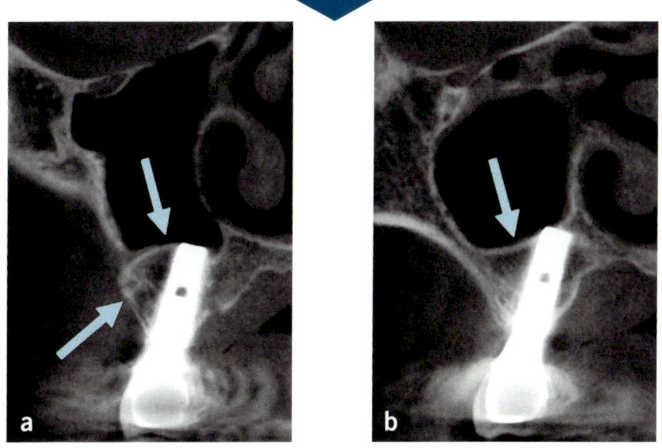


Fig 4-100 (a and b) Postoperative CT images at 2 years.

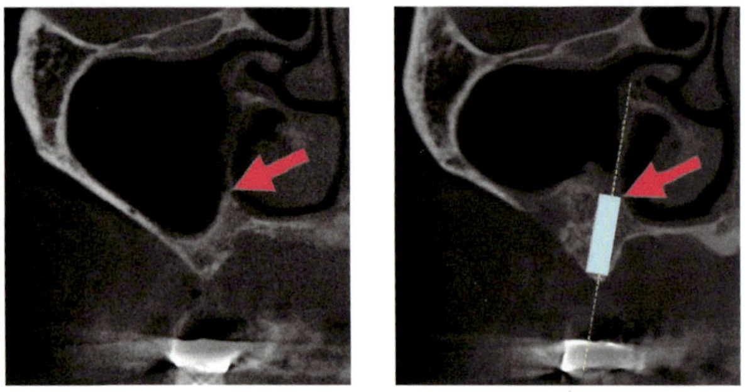

**Figs 4-101 and 4-102** CT images of the maxillary sinus.

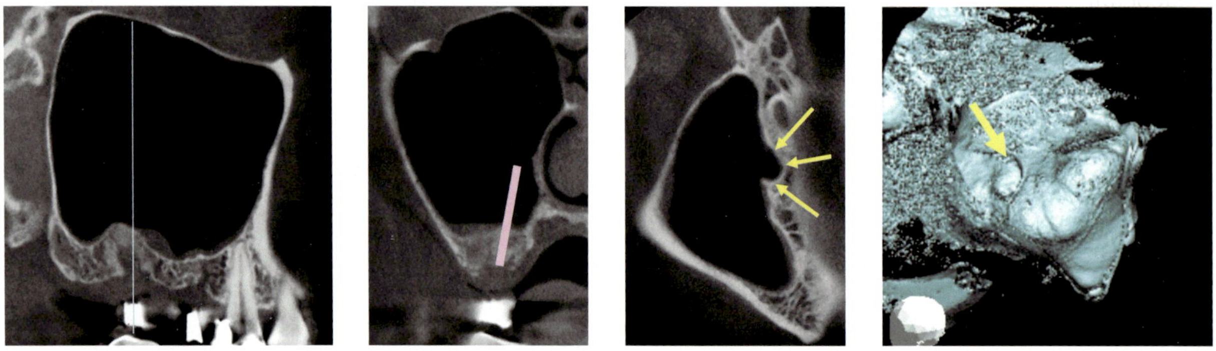

**Figs 4-103 to 4-106** Preoperative CT images.

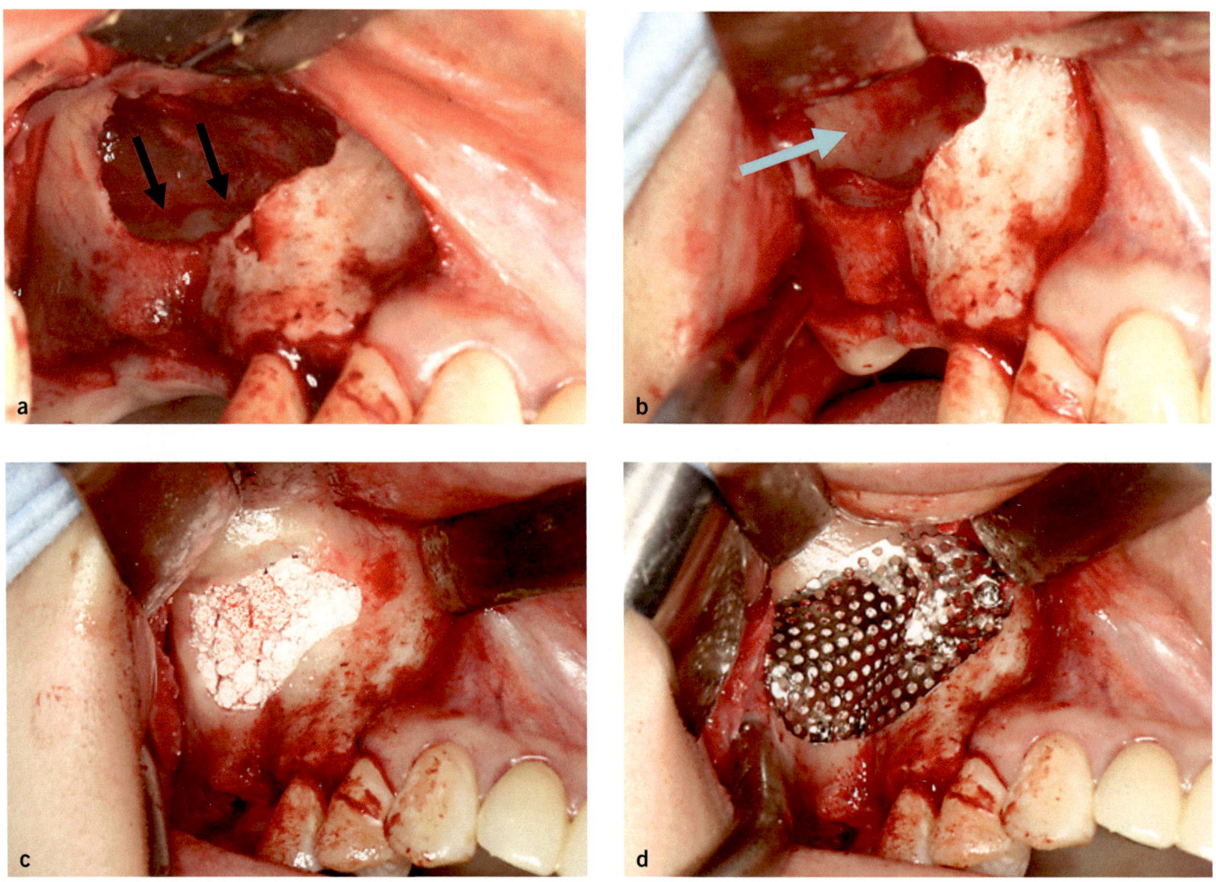

**Fig 4-107** (a to d) Intraoperative intraoral views.

tional cusp of the opposing tooth, the implant apex is often directed toward the medial wall of the maxillary sinus (yellow dotted line on Fig 4-102). Therefore, sufficient sinus membrane elevation is extremely important to accommodate the implant (red arrows on Figs 4-101 and 4-102). Because the bone surface of the medial wall is frequently uneven, the membrane must be dissected very carefully. Use horizon-

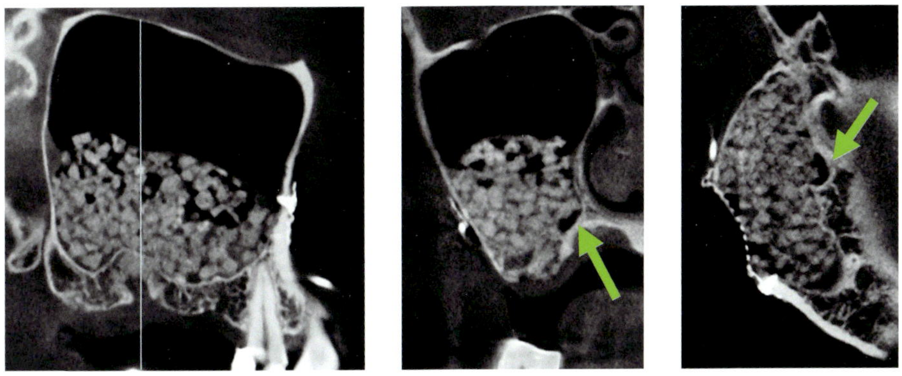

**Figs 4-108 to 4-110** Postoperative CT images.

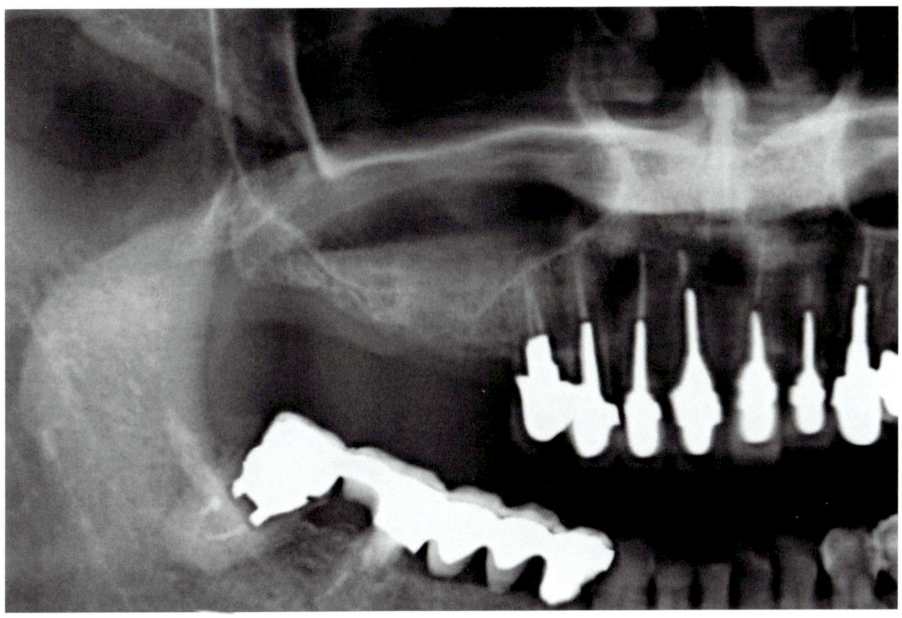

**Fig 4-111** Preoperative panoramic image.

tal cross-sectional and volume rendering CT images to evaluate the bone morphology of the medial wall.

This patient was referred for implant placements at positions 16 and 17. The planned implant sites presented with lack of bone height and required a sinus floor elevation (Fig 4-103). Based on the insertion direction of the implant at position 17 (pink line on Fig 4-104), bone augmentation at the medial wall was considered necessary. Preoperative CT imaging revealed a bone with concave shape in the medial wall (yellow arrows on Figs 4-105 and 4-106).

> **! Key Point**
>
> Ensure sufficient elevation of the sinus membrane in the medial and posterior regions of the maxillary sinus.

Intraoral views during the surgery are shown (Fig 4-107). After fully elevating the sinus membrane in the medial region (black arrows on Fig 4-107a) and posterior region (blue arrow on Fig 4-107b) of the maxillary sinus, the space was filled with β-TCP granules and closed with a titanium mesh over the lateral window (Fig 4-107d).

As can be seen on the CT images immediately after surgery, the β-TCP granules were surrounded by some air bubbles (Figs 4-108 to 4-110). The sinus membrane in the medial region was fully elevated (green arrow on Figs 4-109 and 4-100).

## Resorption of augmented bone beside the medial wall

Resorption of the augmented area beside the medial wall may occur despite sufficient elevation of the sinus membrane. The cause has not yet been elucidated. It seems to occur more often in cases with a depression shape of the medial wall beneath the nasal floor before the surgery.

This patient with loss of teeth 15 to 17 was treated with sinus floor elevation (Fig 4-111). Preoperative

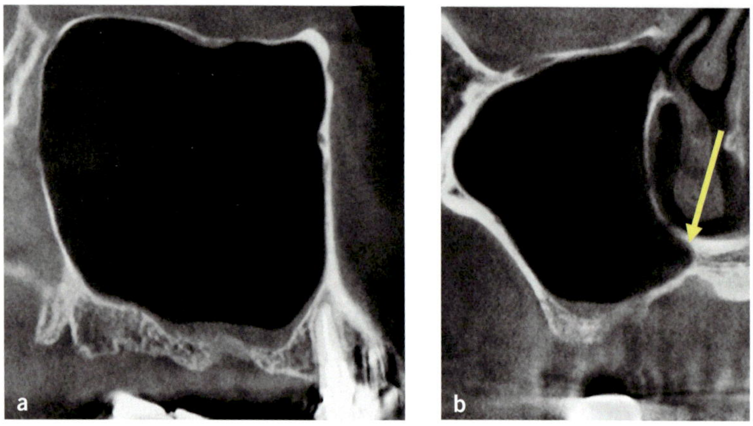


**Fig 4-112** (a and b) Preoperative CT images.

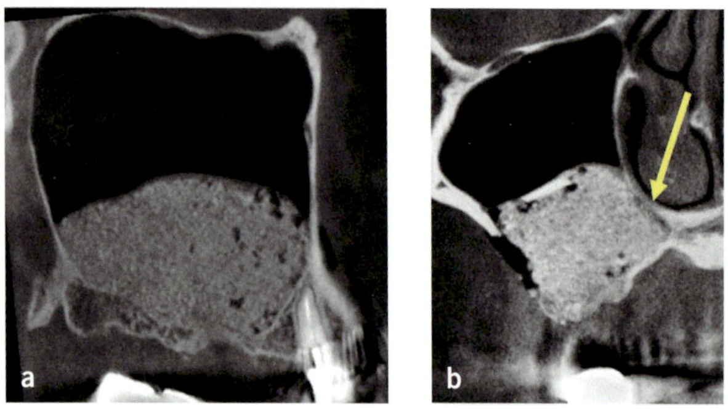


**Fig 4-113** (a and b) CT images immediately after the surgery.

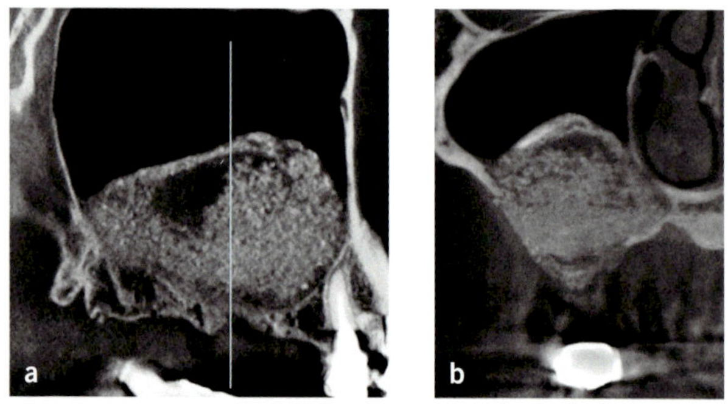


**Fig 4-114** (a and b) CT images 3 months after the surgery.

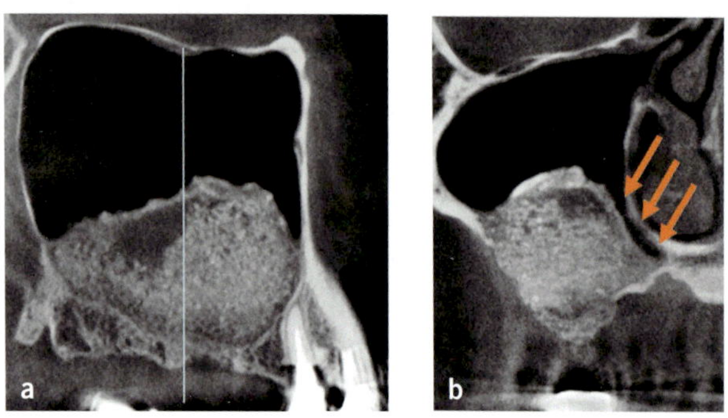


**Fig 4-115** (a and b) CT images at 6 months.

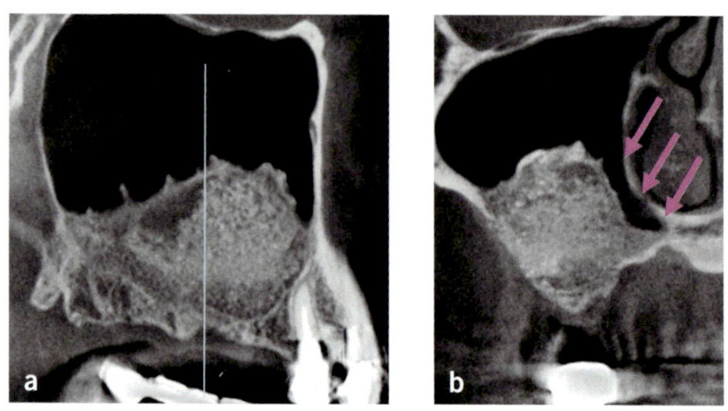


**Fig 4-116** (a and b) CT images at 9 months.

CT scans indicated downward development of the maxillary sinus and an internal concave surface of the medial wall beneath the nasal floor (Fig 4-112a and yellow arrow on Fig 4-112b).

A CT image taken immediately after surgery showed a sufficient amount of β-TCP granules beside the medial wall of the maxillary sinus (Fig 4-113a, and yellow arrow on Fig 4-113b).

Three months after surgery, there was no swelling of the sinus membrane and the β-TCP granules were observed at the original position (Fig 4-114). At 6 months, a slight reduction of the augmented volume was observed with a gap produced between the newly formed sinus floor and the medial wall of the sinus cavity (Fig 4-115a, and orange arrows on Fig 4-115b). At 9 months, the gap inside the augmented space was larger than that observed at 6 months (Fig 4-116a, and pink arrows on Fig 4-116b).

Implants were placed 1 year after the surgery (Figs 4-117 and 4-118). The insertion angle was adjusted to prevent the implant apex from penetrating the elevated sinus floor (green arrow on Fig 4-118a). The gap inside the augmented space continued to grow gradually even after implant placement. After 2.5 years of sinus floor elevation, the gap almost reached the implant apex (blue arrows on Fig 4-118d).

In the region where β-TCP granules were placed, on the other hand, cortical and cancellous bone-like radiopacities were observed at the 2-year postoperative mark and a radiopaque line was found at the lateral window (yellow arrows on Fig 4-118c). The prognosis of the gap inside the augmented area is unknown and follow-up by CT scanning will be important.

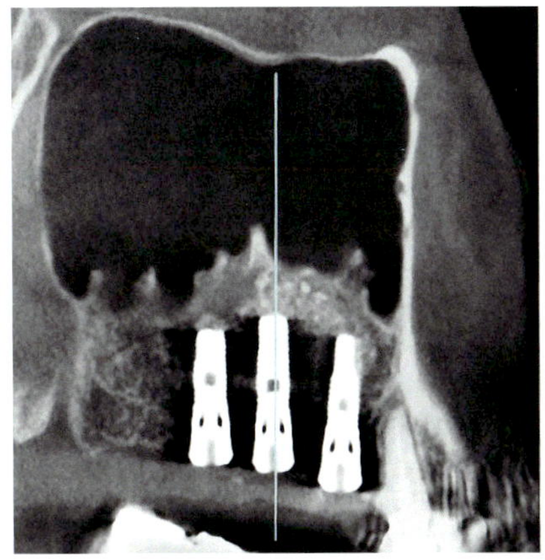

**Fig 4-117** CT images of the implants immediately after placement.

## A perforated sinus membrane

If the sinus membrane is perforated during sinus floor elevation and left untreated, bone substitutes may enter into the sinus cavity through the perforation and result in sinusitis. A full understanding of how to deal with membrane perforation is important.

### Recovery using the bone plate of the lateral window

This patient with loss of teeth 24 to 27 was referred for implant treatment. There was no swelling of the sinus membrane, but there were two residual roots (26 and 27) (Fig 4-119, and yellow arrows on Figs 4-120 a and c). The sinus membrane seemed to be in direct contact with these residual roots.

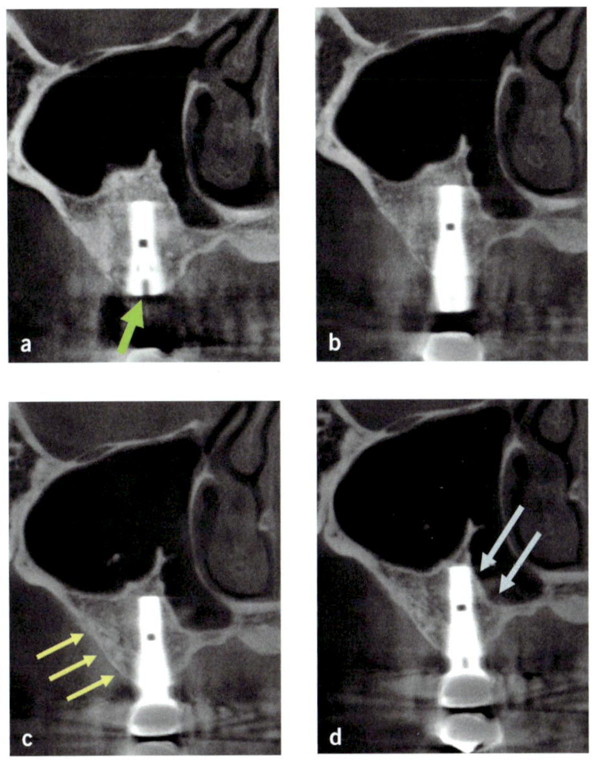

**Fig 4-118** (a to d) CT images at 1, 1.5, 2, and 2.5 years.

> **! Key Point**
>
> Cover the perforation with the bone plate of the lateral window.

During dissection of the sinus membrane, perforations occurred at locations close to the residual roots (black arrows on Fig 4-121a). The bone plate of the lateral window was separated from the sinus membrane (blue arrow on Fig 4-121b) and placed over the perforation (green arrow on Fig 4-121c). The up and down movements of the sinus membrane by breathing was recovered by the coverage of the perforation, and then β-TCP granules were placed under the elevated sinus membrane (Fig 4-121d).

CT images taken immediately after surgery, and at 3 and 10 months after surgery, are shown (Fig 4-122). The horizontal shadow on the CT image immediately after surgery (yellow arrow on Fig 4-122a) reveals that the blood and saline solution entered into the sinus cavity through the perforations of the sinus membrane (because the CT scan was performed in a sitting position). The bone plate of the lateral window was

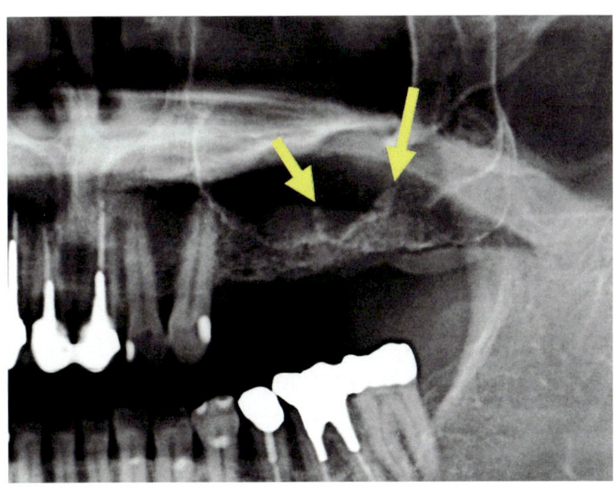

**Fig 4-119** Panoramic view before the corrective surgery.

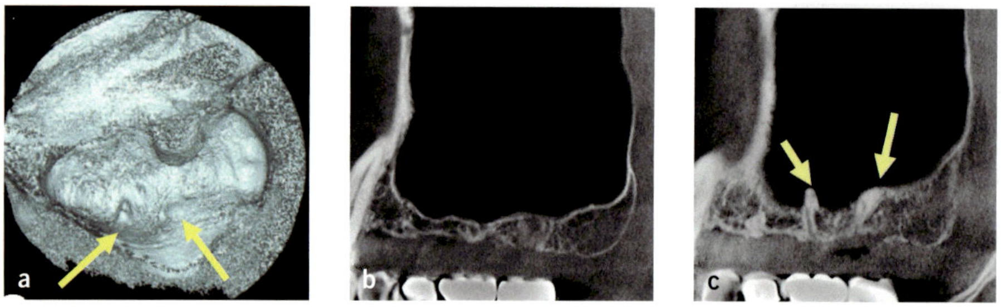


**Fig 4-120** (a to c) CT images showing residual roots.

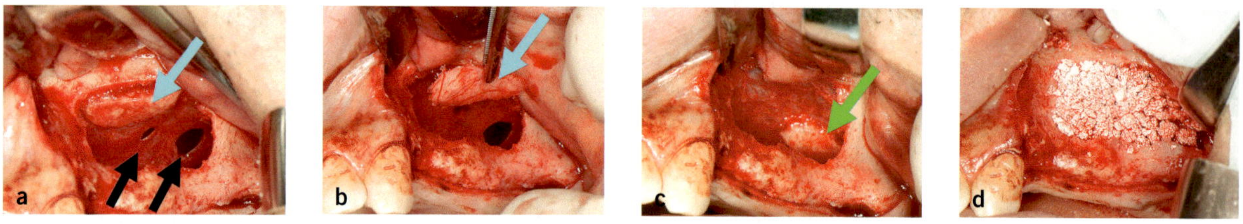


**Fig 4-121** (a to d) Intraoperative intraoral views.

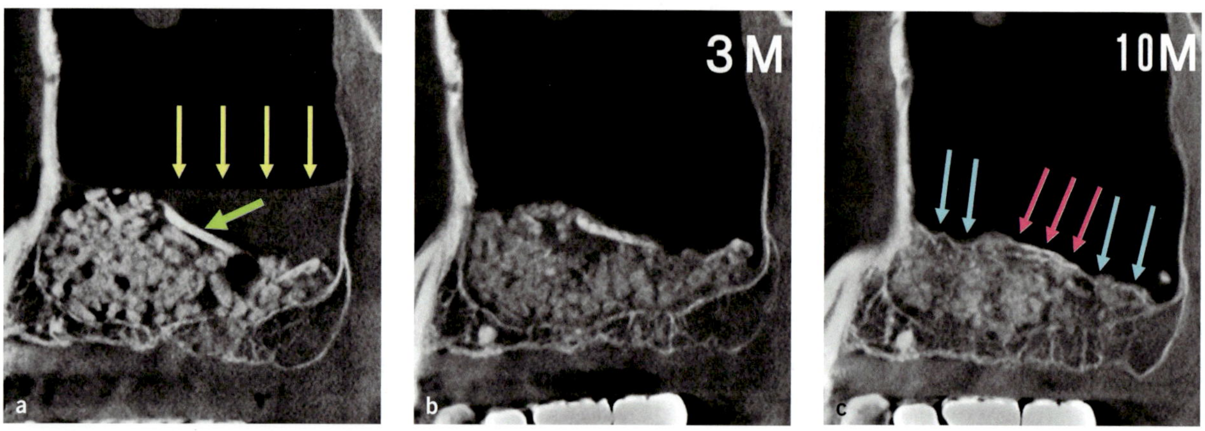


**Fig 4-122** (a to c) CT images immediately after the surgery and at 3 and 10 months.

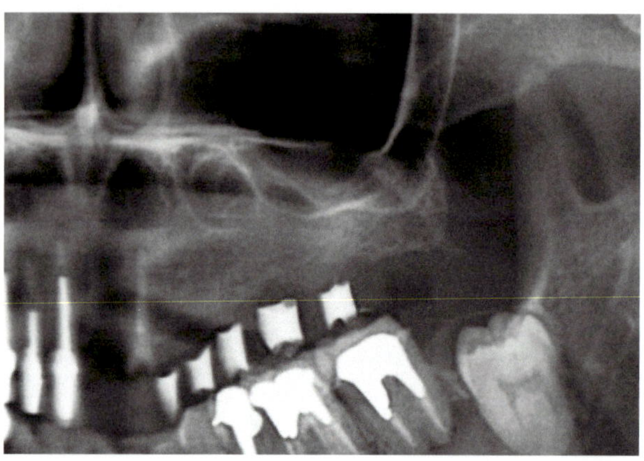

**Fig 4-123** Preoperative panoramic view.

shown as a radiopacity (green arrow on Fig 4-122a) and no dislocation of β-TCP granules into the sinus cavity was observed. Three months after surgery, the β-TCP granule size became slightly smaller and there was some resorption of the bone plate of the lateral window (Fig 4-122b). The CT image taken 10 months after surgery reveals that the bone plate of the lateral window placed over the perforations was almost completely resorbed (red arrows on Fig 4-122c) and the boundary between the bone of the lateral window and the radiopaque line of the newly formed sinus floor (blue arrows on Fig 4-122c) is unclear. There is no swelling of the sinus membrane, and the β-TCP granules further reduced in size and appeared to have integrated with the lateral window bone.

## Recovery using a collagen membrane

A patient had undergone sinus floor elevation with iliac bone marrow particulates at the Department of Oral Surgery of a university hospital, but was unable to revisit the original hospital. A panoramic view was obtained by the author's team (Fig 4-123). Preoperative CT scans were also taken (Figs 4-124 to 4-129). There was a bony projection in the anterior area (red arrow on Fig 4-124) and soft tissue invasion beneath the bony projection (yellow arrow

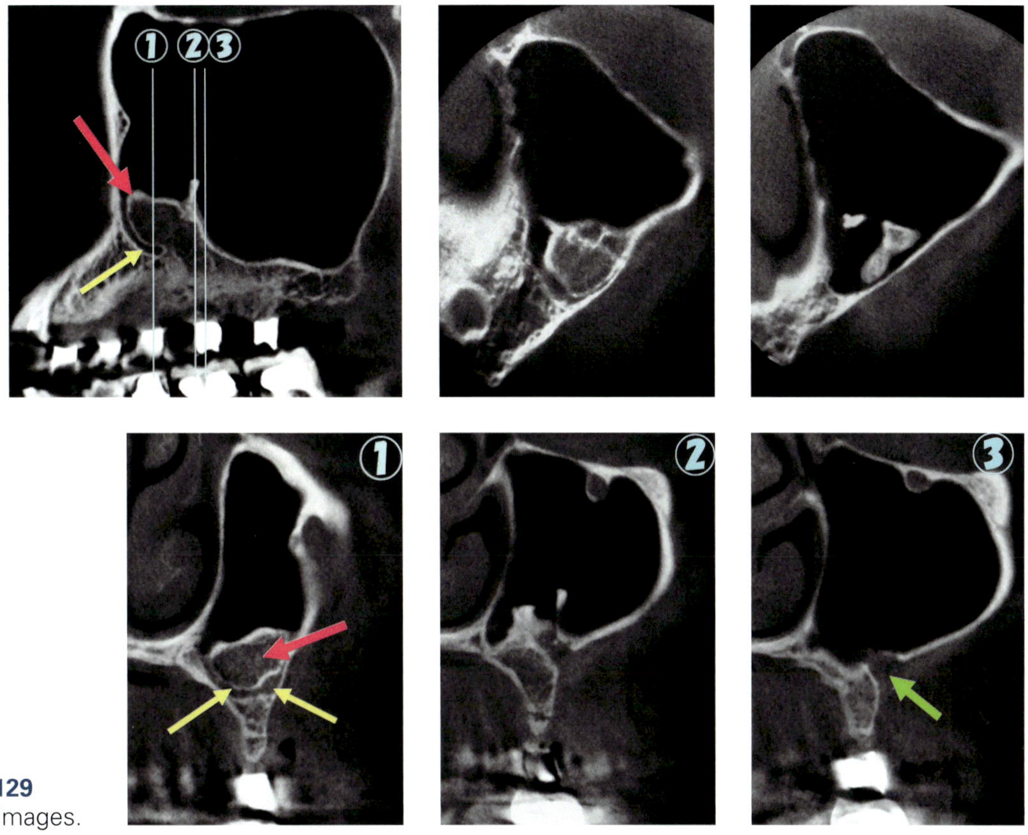


**Figs 4-124 to 4-129**
Preoperative CT images.

on Fig 4-124), which indicated that implant placement in this region was too risky. Further, several projections toward the maxillary sinus (Fig 4-128) and a bone defect (green arrow on Fig 4-129) were discovered on the CT images.

Because the patient strongly desired implant treatment, removal of the bony projection and sinus floor elevation using β-TCP granules were provided again.

For the bone defect on the buccal aspect, a sharp incision of soft tissue was made using a surgical knife (yellow arrow on Fig 4-130a) and the mucoperiosteal flap was reflected with careful attention to avoid membrane perforation (Fig 4-130b). Osteotomy to create the lateral window was made using a diamond round bur. Osteotomy was also made to the base of the bony projection (black arrows on Fig 4-130c). Using a small scalpel (Martin), the maxillary sinus membrane was dissected from the posterior and superior areas of the projection (Fig 4-130d).

The bony projection was split, and the sinus membrane in the anterior region was elevated while removing the bony projection, which resulted in perforations of the sinus membrane (Figs 4-130e to 4-130g, and yellow arrows on Fig 4-130h).

A collagen membrane (Terdarmis with no silicon membrane), trimmed to the proper shape, was placed to cover the perforations, and then β-TCP granules were placed into the space (Figs 4-130i and 4-130j). After covering the lateral window with a titanium mesh (Fig 4-130k), a Penrose drain was inserted through the vertical incision (black arrow on Fig 4-130l) and fixed by a stitch.

> **! Key Point**
>
> As described in a later section, the author makes it a rule to close the lateral window with a titanium mesh. This better stabilizes the β-TCP granules and facilitates insertion of a drain, and thus alleviates the postoperative facial swelling.

A panoramic radiograph and CT images were obtained immediately after surgery (Figs 4-131 and 4-132). The Penrose drain is observed as a radioopacity (green arrows). The collagen membrane is observed above the augmented region (yellow arrows on Fig 4-132), and no β-TCP granules have shifted into the sinus cavity.

As shown on the CT images 3 months after surgery (Fig 4-133), the sinus membrane presented slight swelling but there was no dislocation of β-TCP granules into the sinus cavity.

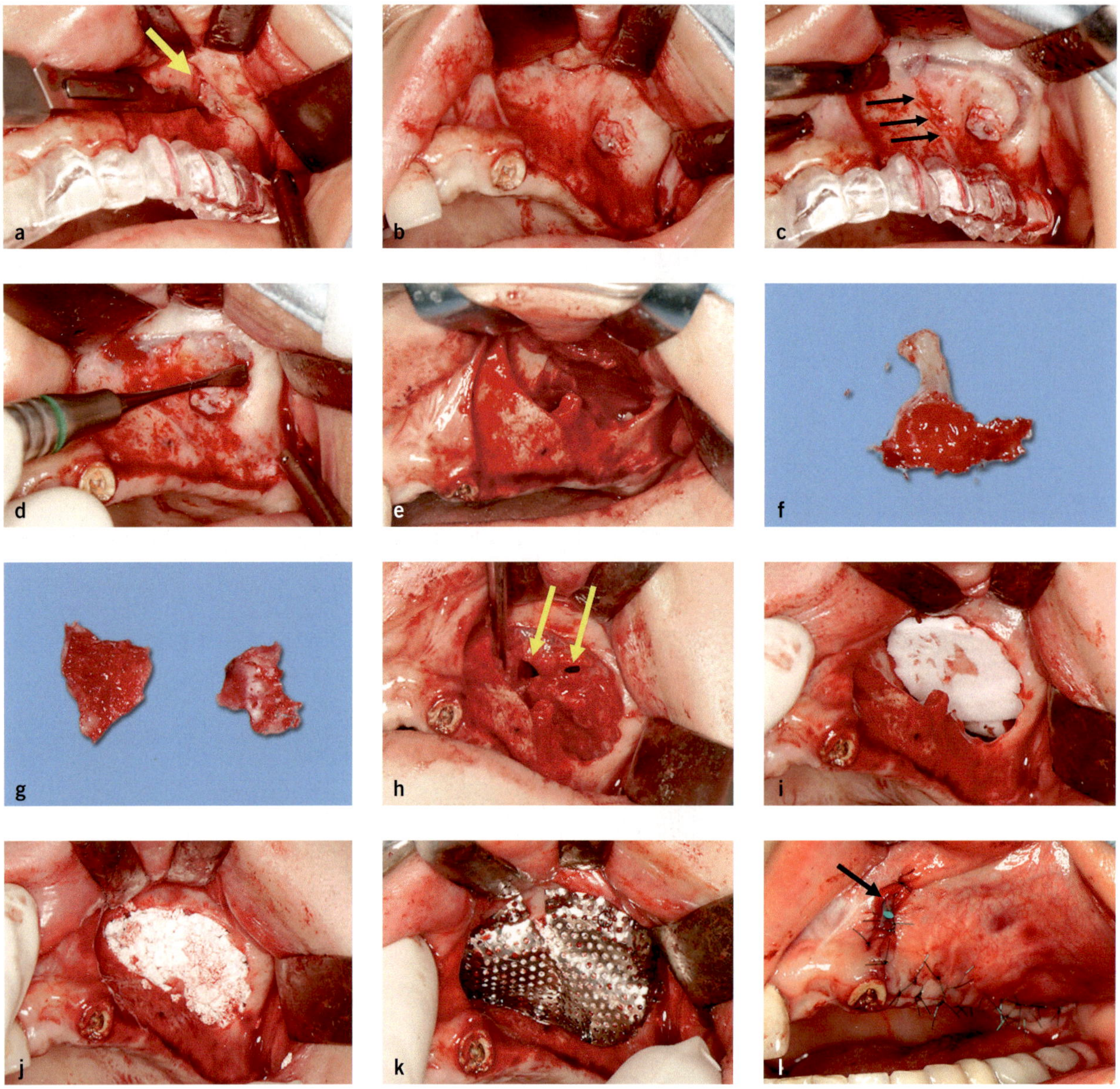


**Fig 4-130** (a to l) Intraoperative intraoral views.

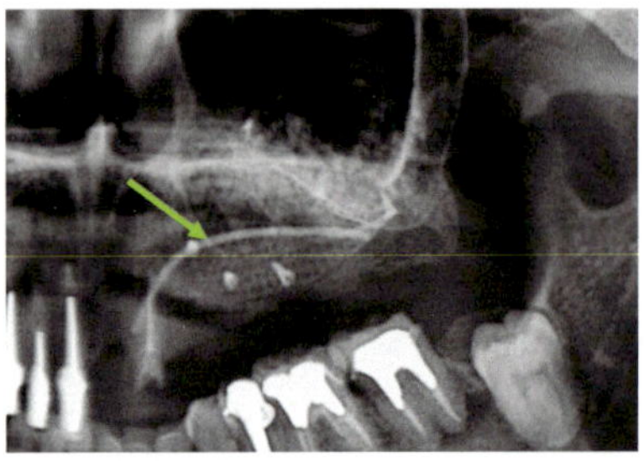

**Fig 4-131** Panoramic view immediately after the surgery.

CT images were obtained 10 months after surgery (Fig 4-134). On the sagittal CT image, no swelling of the sinus membrane is observed and the collagen membrane used to cover the perforation has disappeared. The β-TCP granule size became smaller and the cortical-bone–like line indicating the newly formed sinus floor was seen. The original sinus floor became unclear (pink arrows on Fig 4-134a). The buccolingual CT image showed radiopaque lines at the lateral window and the newly formed sinus floor (yellow arrows on Figs 4-134b and c).

The titanium mesh was removed 1 year after the surgery, and implants were placed (Figs 4-135). To correct the reduced buccolingual width of the alveolar ridge, guided bone regeneration (GBR) was performed simultaneously with implant placement.

A postoperative panoramic radiograph and further buccolingual CT images were obtained (Figs 4-136 and 4-137). Thus, re-performing sinus floor elevation provided the environment to accommodate longer implants.

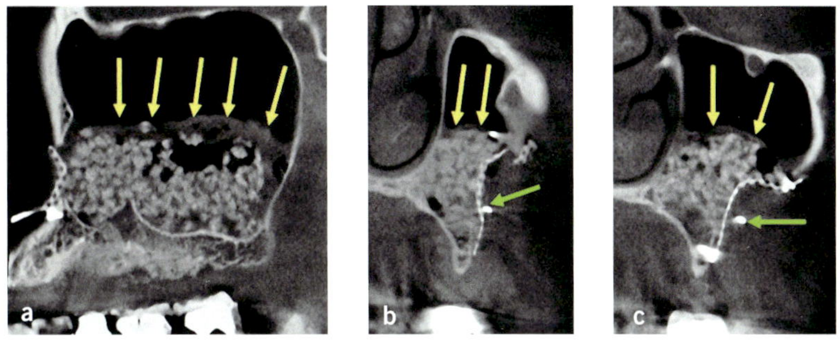

**Fig 4-132** (a to c) CT images immediately after the surgery.

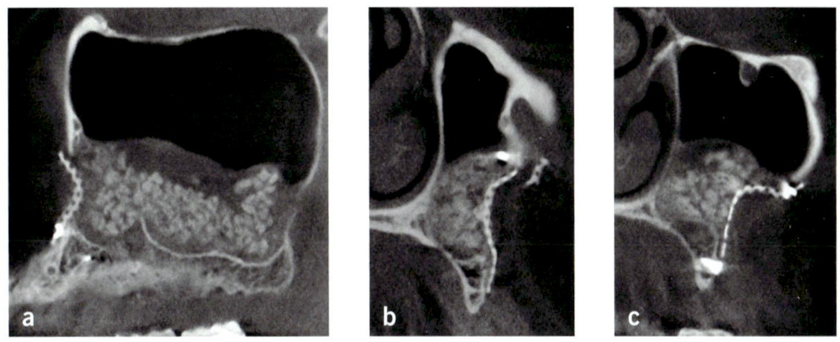

**Fig 4-133** (a to c) CT images 3 months after the surgery.

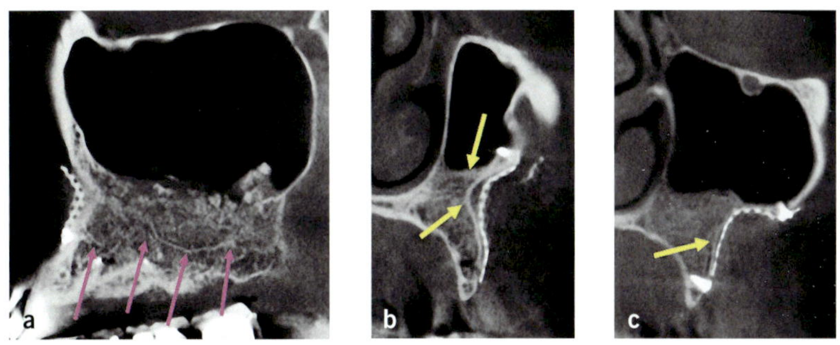

**Fig 4-134** (a to c) CT images 10 months after the surgery.

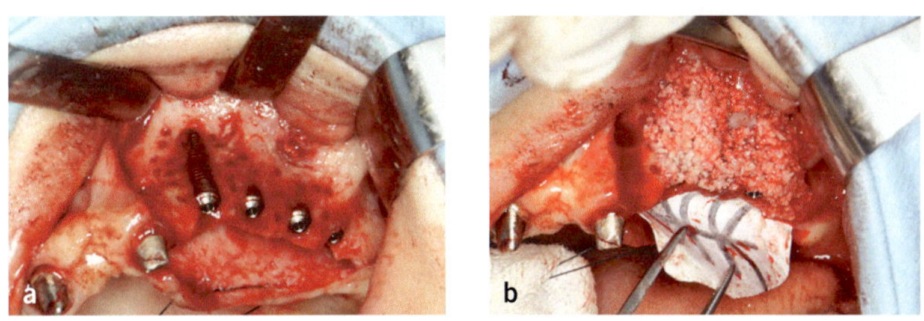

**Fig 4-135** (a and b) Intraoral views 1 year after sinus floor elevation by the lateral window technique.

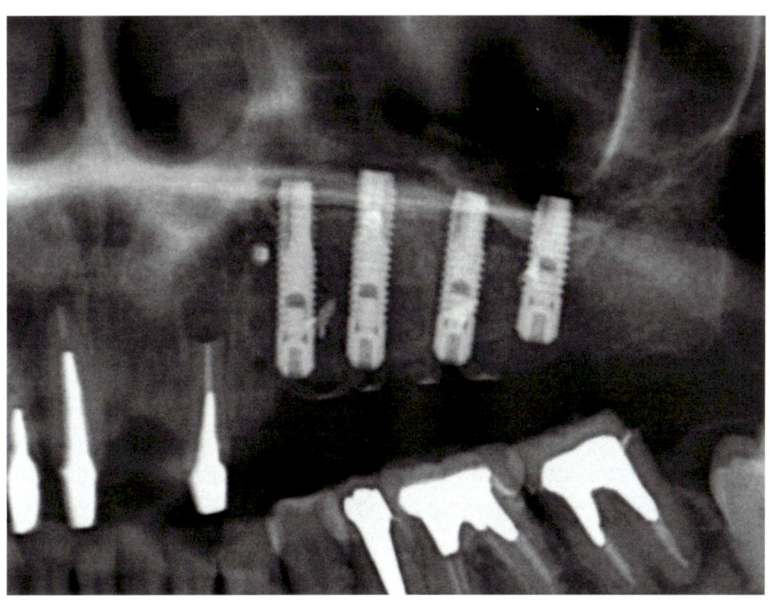

**Fig 4-136** Panoramic view immediately after implant placement and simultaneous GBR.

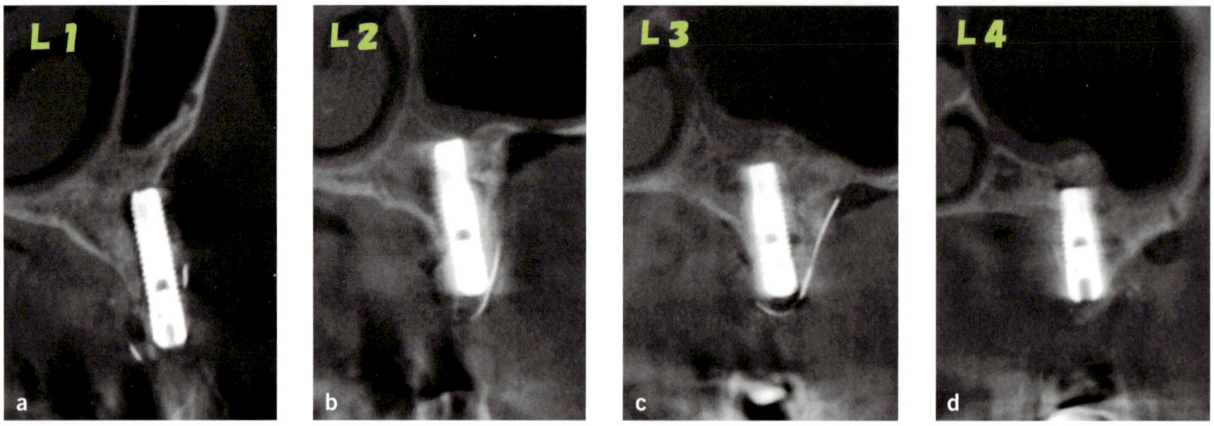


**Fig 4-137** (a to d) CT images immediately after implant placement and simultaneous GBR.

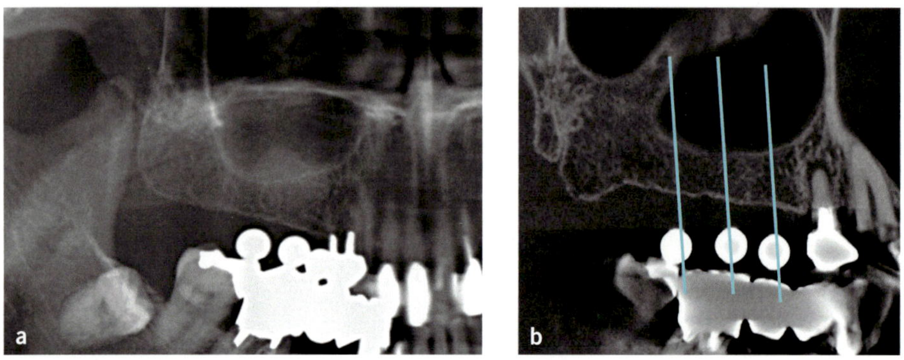


**Fig 4-138** (a and b) Panoramic views before the surgery.

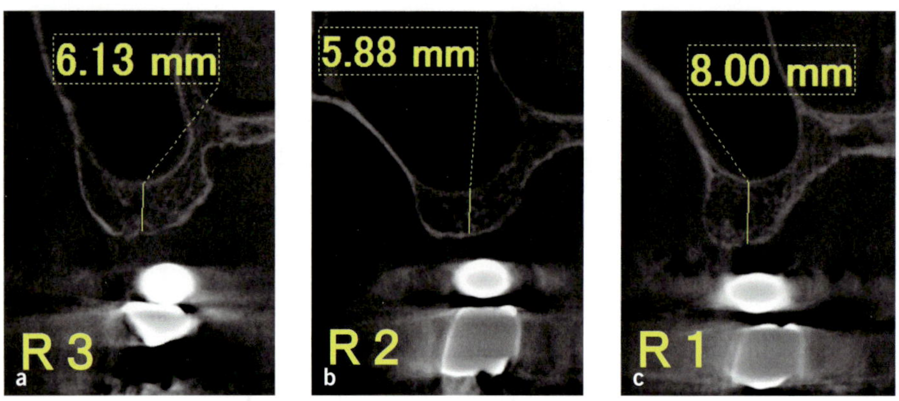


**Fig 4-139** (a to c) CT images views before the surgery.

## How safe is implant placement with simultaneous sinus floor elevation?

In recent years, implant placement with simultaneous sinus floor elevation has gained popularity, in order to decrease surgical invasiveness and shorten the treatment period. However, it is impossible to determine clinically whether the fixture has achieved osseointegration in the augmented region, and there exists the possibility that the implant has osseointegrated only with native bone. Such was the case with the patient presented in this section, who had received implant placement simultaneously with sinus floor elevation.

> **! Key Point**
>
> As a result of encountering this case, the author has made it a rule not to place implants simultaneously with sinus floor elevation unless sufficient primary stability is first confirmed.

### Surgical procedure: implant placement and sinus floor elevation

The patient presented with loss of teeth 15 to 17. Because the ridge height was over 5 mm, implants were placed simultaneously with sinus floor elevation (Figs 4-138 and 4-139).

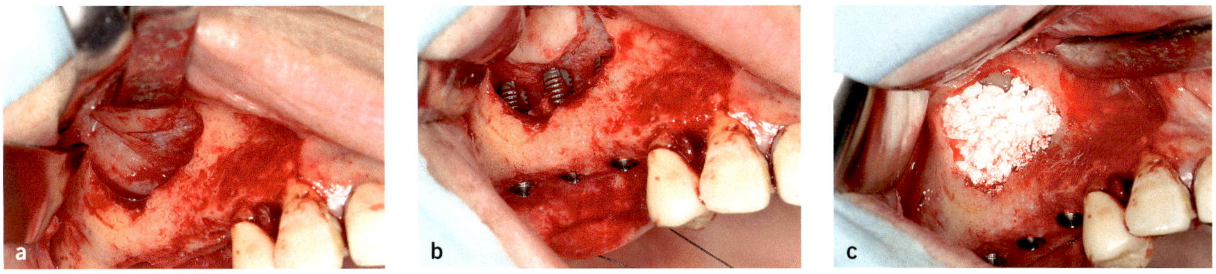

**Fig 4-140** (a to c) Intraoperative intraoral views.

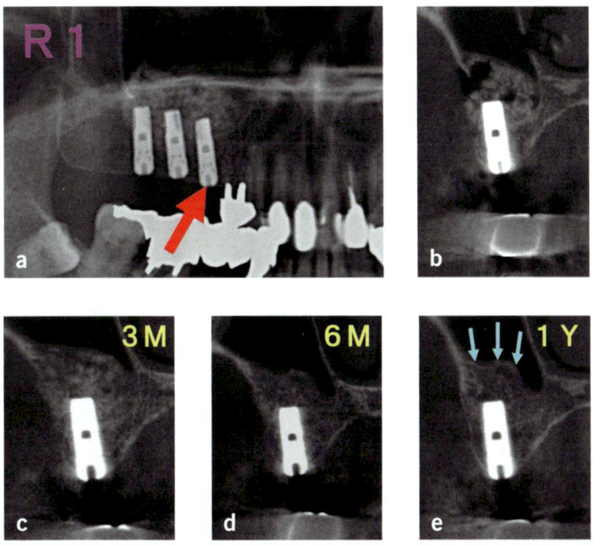


**Fig 4-141** (a and b) R1: panoramic view and CT image immediately after surgery, and (c to e) CT images 3, 6, and 12 months after surgery.

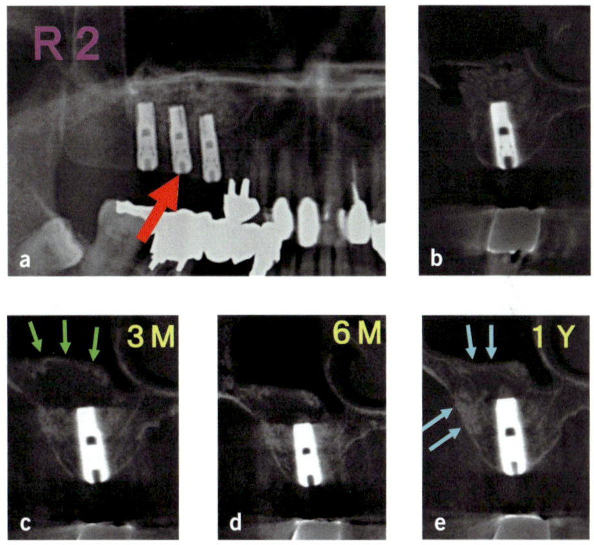


**Fig 4-142** (a and b) R2: panoramic view and CT image immediately after surgery, and (c to e) CT images 3, 6, and 12 months after surgery.

Using the standard procedure, the maxillary sinus membrane was elevated, three implants were placed, and the space was then filled with β-TCP granules (Fig 4-140).

In contrast to the good primary stability of implant R1, the remaining two implants (R2 and R3) showed unfavorable primary stability and had to be stabilized by densely packing β-TCP granules around them. As described later, the maxillary sinus membrane developed swelling at 1 week after surgery, which led to dislodging of β-TCP granules. Unfortunately, the author, at the time of the treatment of this patient, was unaware of the negative impact of the postoperative membrane swelling. In retrospect, the implant stability of R2 and R3 must have been lost 1 week after the placement.

## Postoperative imaging

Postoperative images of R1 are shown (Fig 4-141). Six months after surgery, the β-TCP granules became decreased in size. One year after surgery the radiopaque line of the newly formed sinus floor was visible (blue arrows on Fig 4-141e).

Postoperative images of R2 are shown next (Fig 4-142). The CT image taken immediately after surgery demonstrates the presence of dense β-TCP granules around the implant. Three months after, the β-TCP granules, which originally surrounded the implant apex, have shifted upward (green arrows on Fig 4-142c). The granules must have been dislodged by swelling of the maxillary sinus membrane that developed 1 week after surgery. One year after surgery, the radiopaque lines at the lateral window and the newly formed sinus floor can be seen (blue arrows on Fig 4-142e).

Finally, postoperative images of R3 are shown (Fig 4-143). Similar to the case of implant R2, densely packed β-TCP granules are observed around the implant immediately after surgery. One year after surgery, the radiopaque line of the newly formed sinus floor can be seen (blue arrows on Fig 4-143e), and the prognosis was favorable.

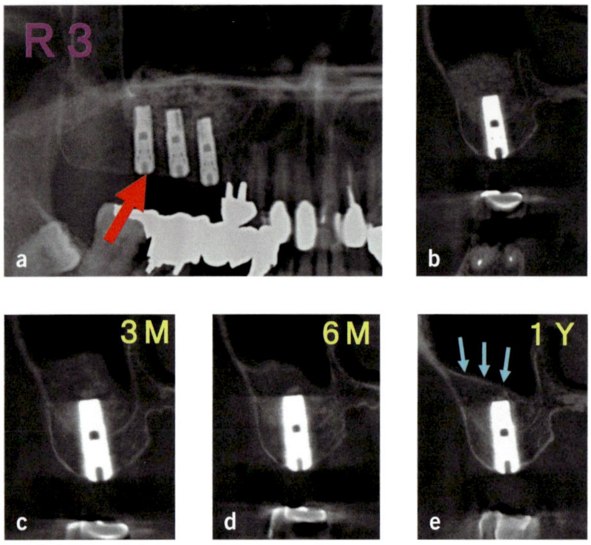


**Fig 4-143** (a and b) R3: panoramic view and CT image immediately after surgery, and (c to e) CT images 3, 6, and 12 months after surgery.

> **! Key Point**
>
> Implant placement at the same time as sinus floor elevation cannot provide any assurance that the fixture in the augmented region can achieve osseointegration.

> **! Key Point**
>
> There may be individual variability, at a genetic level, in osteogenic capability. Prognosis of sinus floor elevation may be affected by the osteogenic capability of each individual patient.

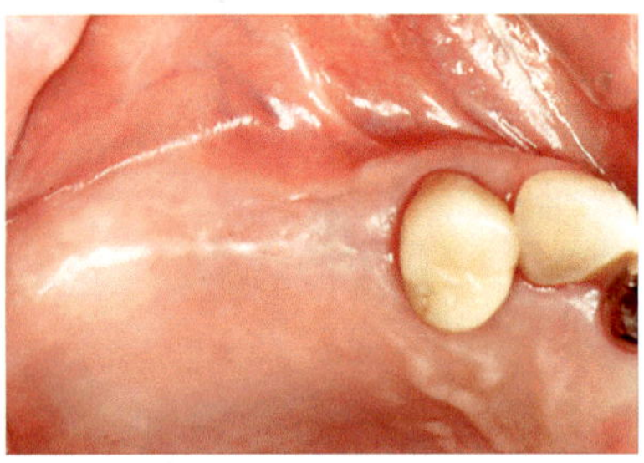

**Fig 4-144** No visible gingival inflammation.

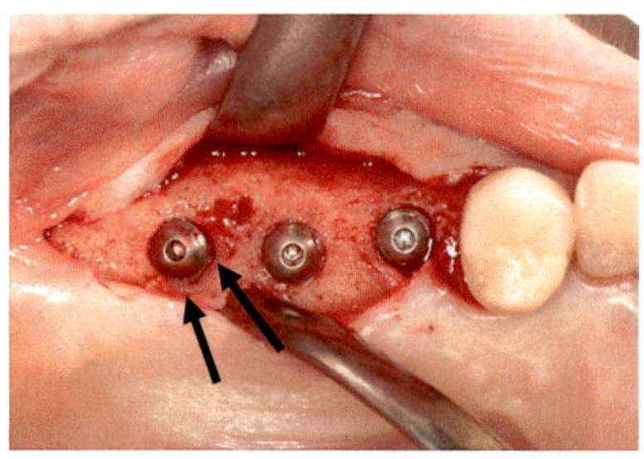

**Fig 4-145** R3 shows osseointegration failure.

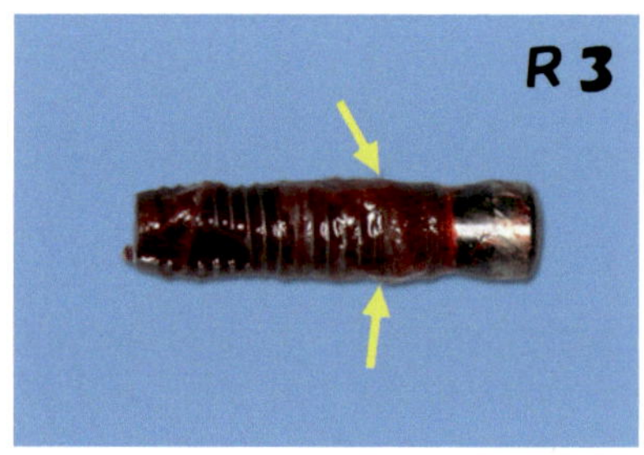


**Fig 4-146** R3 removed.

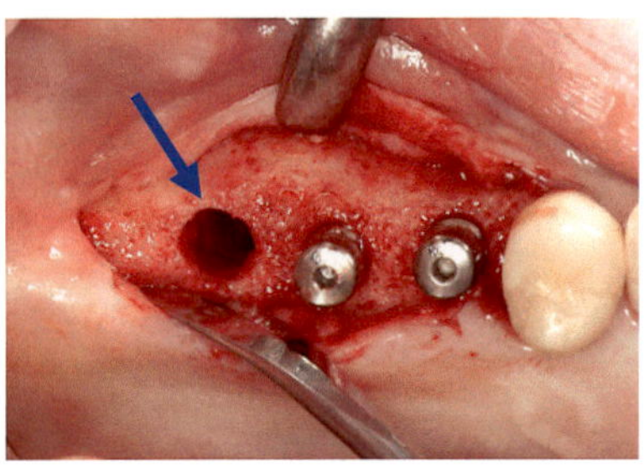

**Fig 4-147** R3 socket after removal.

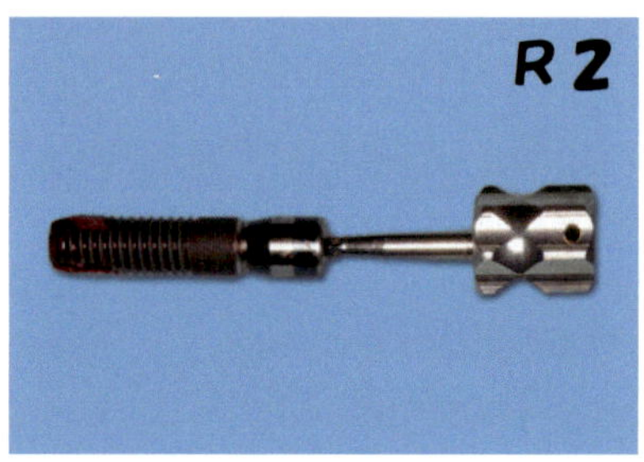


**Fig 4-148** R2 removed.

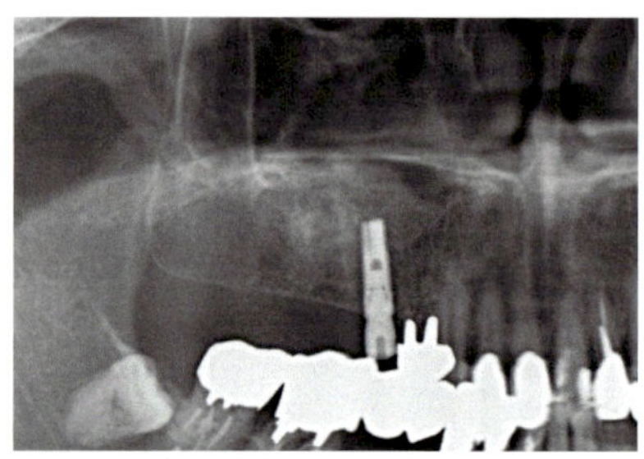

**Fig 4-149** Panoramic view after the second surgery.

## Second surgery: removal and re-implantation

The postoperative clinical course was uneventful and there was no sign of gingival inflammation (Fig 4-144). Therefore, the second surgery was performed 1 year after implant placement. Implant R3 presented osseointegration failure, with soft tissue at its mesial and palatal aspects (black arrows on Fig 4-145). The surface of the removed implant was covered with soft tissue (yellow arrows on Fig 4-146). However, no significant crestal bone defect was observed at the margin of the implant socket (blue arrow on Fig 4-147).

The cover screws of implants R1 and R2 were replaced with healing abutments. During abutment connection no implant mobility was detected. However, the bone quality was insufficiently dense and there was a concern as to whether these implants could withstand functional loads. Therefore, osseointegration of the two implants was evaluated by applying a load. When a load was applied to implant

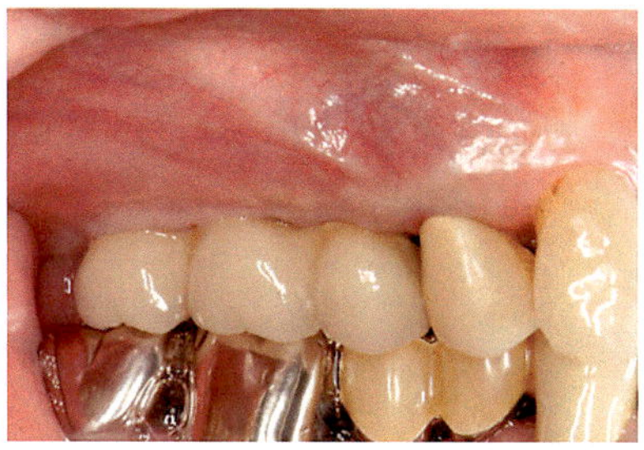

**Fig 4-150** (left) Intraoral view 16 months after the final restoration.

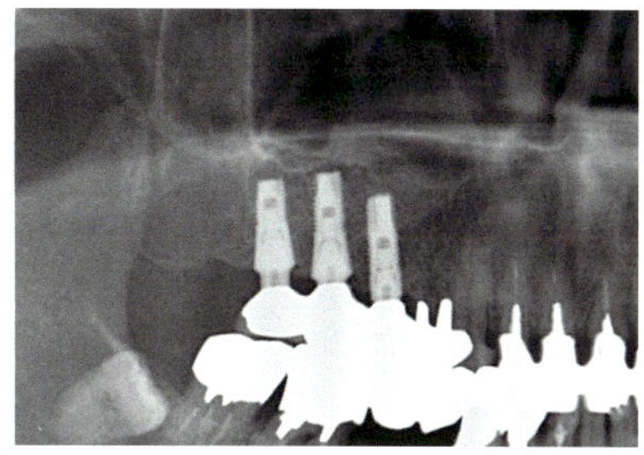

**Fig 4-151** (right) Panoramic view 16 months after the final restoration.

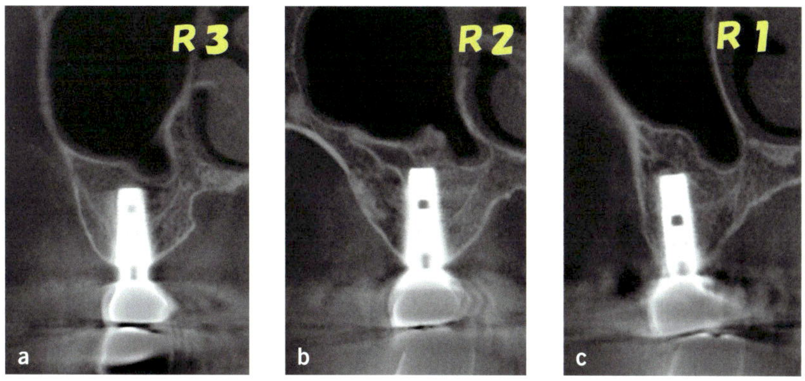


**Fig 4-152** (a to c) CT images 16 months after the final restoration.

R2 via the healing abutment, R2 gradually began to present mobility, so it was removed too (Fig 4-148). Discovered on the fixture surface was a small amount of residual β-TCP granules with almost no granulation tissue. Hard tissue was present at the apex of the implant socket and there was no communication with the maxillary sinus cavity.

Implant R2 appeared to have osseointegrated only with the native bone, which was the reason that no mobility was detected during healing abutment connection. The quality of the native bone was not dense enough, so the load applied via the healing abutment destroyed the osseointegration (Fig 4–148). This observation suggested that, in the augmented area, a layer of soft tissue was formed around the fixture instead of osseointegration, indicating that an implant placement simultaneously with sinus floor elevation cannot provide any assurance that the fixture in the augmented region can achieve osseointegration. When the primary stability is inadequate, simultaneous implant placement should be avoided for safety reasons.

In this patient, re-implantation took place 6 months after the removal of R2 and R3. The two new implants were allowed to heal for 5 months. Fortunately the new implants achieved osseointegration, but the treatment period exceeded the original schedule by about a year.

Figures 4-150 to 4-152 are the intraoral view, panoramic radiograph and CT images 16 months after the final restoration (2 years after re-implantation and 3.5 years after sinus floor elevation). There was no sign of gingival inflammation and the clinical course looked uneventful. The radiopacity of the augmented region, or the new bone formed on β-TCP granules, was comparable to that of native bone. This finding indicates that the newly formed bone on a β-TCP scaffold may have the same quality as the native bone. In other words, there may be individual variability, at a genetic level, in the osteogenic capability, and the prognosis of sinus floor elevation may be affected by the osteogenic capability of each individual patient.

## 4.3 The postoperative stage

### Introduction

In the hospital where the author worked prior to establishing a private clinic, although helical CT images were obtained as part of the preoperative examination process for sinus floor elevation, none were taken after the surgery because of the high dose of radiation inherent in such scans.

During his time at the hospital, the author encountered a patient who presented with abnormal gingival swelling 1 week after surgery, extending from the vertical incision area to the buccogingival transition zone; this occurred despite the fact that facial swelling had disappeared. The patient had been treated with sinus floor elevation and simultaneous guided bone regeneration (GBR). Upon examination, something hard was felt immediately beneath the swollen gingiva.

At 2 weeks after the surgery, being surprised by purulence from the vertical incision area, the author obtained an urgent CT scan. Severe swelling of the maxillary sinus membrane was observed and the hard material detected on palpation was identified as β-TCP, which had been used to fill in the space.

> **! Key Point**
>
> Postoperative swelling of the maxillary sinus membrane was revealed only by CT scanning.

At that time, the swelling of the maxillary sinus membrane was considered to have arisen from postoperative infection, and no further probe was made into what caused the dislocation of the β-TCP granules.

When opening his private clinic, the author introduced cone-beam CT (3DX, Morita, Japan). The CBCT equipment can scan an area of 6 cm × 6 cm and provides clear images in spite of an extremely low radiation dose. Originally, the CBCT was expected to detect postoperative infection at an early phase, and a scan was performed of the maxillary sinus membrane 1 week following our surgery.

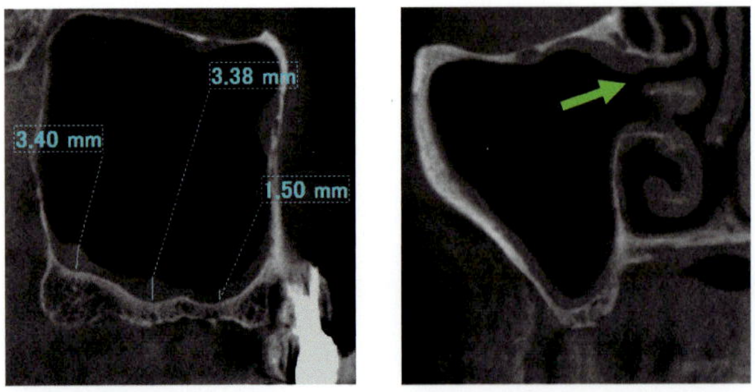


**Fig 4-153** Sample CTs.

The first CT scan taken 1 week after sinus floor elevation revealed significant swelling of the maxillary sinus membrane and dislocation of a small amount of β-TCP through the lateral window, which discouraged the author as he thought it was a postoperative infection. However, the postoperative clinical course of the patient was good. In fact, in subsequent patients who underwent 1-week postoperative CT scans, membrane swelling was observed, more or less, without exception.

Because the postoperative swelling of the maxillary sinus membrane was an unknown phenomenon, the author experienced a sense of trepidation each time when performing the 1-week postoperative CT scan. After observing the same phenomena in 10 consecutive patients, however, it was recognised that the swelling of the maxillary sinus membrane was a natural part of the healing process. In this section, postoperative swelling of the maxillary sinus membrane, including the above finding, is discussed using a series of cases treated by sinus floor elevation.

### Summary of the clinical study

#### Purpose

The aim was to evaluate the maxillary sinus membrane swelling occurring 1 week after sinus floor elevation using CBCT analysis, and assess its influence on the outcome of bone augmentation.

#### Materials and methods

The grafting material was β-TCP (Osferion; Olympus Terumo Biomaterials, Japan). Cone-beam CT was used (3DX; Morita, Japan). CT scans were performed several times for each patient – before, immediately following, 1 week after and >1 month after sinus floor elevation.

#### Subjects

There were 67 patients, with 76 sites in total, recorded over a 4-year period. Sexes: 18 males and 49 females. Ages: 26–70 years (mean 53.7).

#### Postoperative swelling

Maxillary sinus thickening before surgery was *not seen* in 60 cases (78.9%) but was *mild* in 16 cases (21.1%). The ostium remained open in every case (green arrow on Fig 4-153). One-week postoperative CT scans revealed swelling of the maxillary sinus membrane at all 76 sites. Three months after the surgery, the maxillary sinus membrane swelling had disappeared at 74 sites (97.4%).

## Degrees of postoperative sinus membrane swelling

Figure 4-154 shows a summary of the classification used, into three severity groups.

Maxillary sinus membrane swelling occurred 1 week after sinus floor elevation: of type 1 at 13 sites (17.1%), of type 2 at 36 sites (47.4%), and of type 3 at 27 sites (35.5%). Therefore, about 80% of all treated sites presented swelling of the maxillary sinus membrane of over one-third of the volume of the residual maxillary sinus.

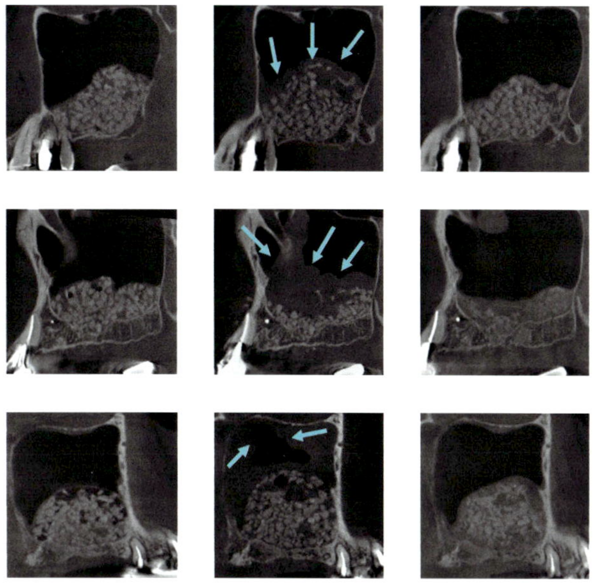

**Fig 4-154** Degrees of postoperative sinus membrane swelling. Top row: type 1 – less than one-third of the remaining sinus cavity; middle row: type 2 – between one-third and two-thirds of the remaining sinus cavity; bottom row: type 3 – more than two-thirds of the remaining sinus cavity. Left column: immediately after surgery; middle column: 1 week post-surgery; right column: 3 months post-surgery.

## Classification of dislocation of grafting material

Dislocation of β-TCP granules from the lateral window was an adverse effect of the membrane swelling. The dislocation of the granules was categorized into three groups, summarized in Figure 4-155 and Table 4-1.

## Brief discussion

The author now always covers the lateral window completely with a titanium mesh or collagen membrane. In the past, the author did not cover the lateral window; so, even for cases treated with simultaneous GBR, the author did not provide complete coverage of the lateral window with a barrier membrane.

Though there are differences in the sample size, granule dislocation was compared by dividing cases into two groups: a group with non- or incomplete coverage of the lateral window (18 sites, 23.7%) and the other group with complete lateral window coverage (58 sites, 76.3%) – see Table 4-1. In the former group, granules remained at the lateral window at 7 sites (38.9%), whereas granule dislocation through the lateral window was observed in about 60%.

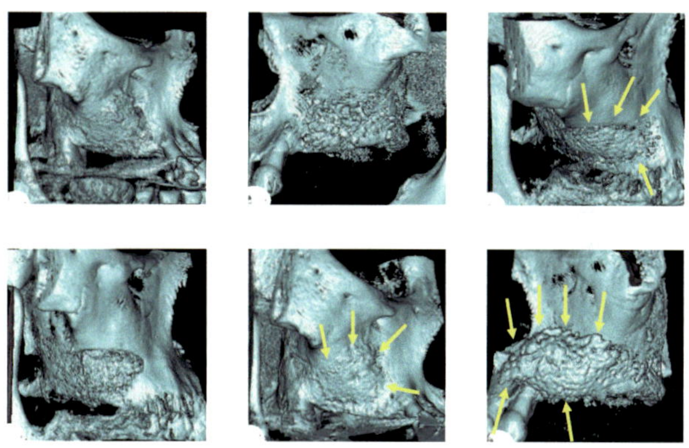

**Fig 4-155** Classification of dislocation of β-TCP granules. Left column: type A – granules remained at the lateral window; middle column: type B – shifted to the adjacent tooth; right column: type C – shifted beyond the adjacent tooth. Top row: immediately after surgery; bottom row: 1 week post-surgery.

**Table 4-1** Lateral window coverage and β-TCP granule dislocation.

| | **Non- or incomplete-coverage** 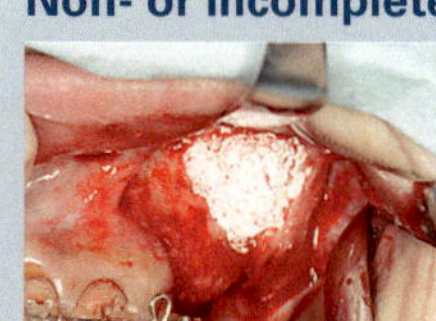 | **Complete coverage** 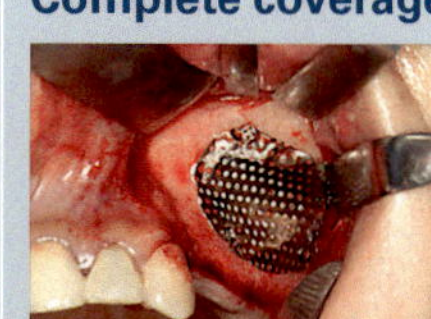 |
|---|---|---|
| All sites | 18 sites (23.7%) | 58 sites (76.3%) |
| Type A (granules remained at the lateral window) | 7 sites (38.9%) | 55 sites (94.8%) |
| Type B (up to the adjacent tooth) | 8 sites (44.4%) | 1 sites (1.7%) |
| Type C (beyond the adjacent tooth) | 3 sites (16.7%) | 2 sites (3.5%) |

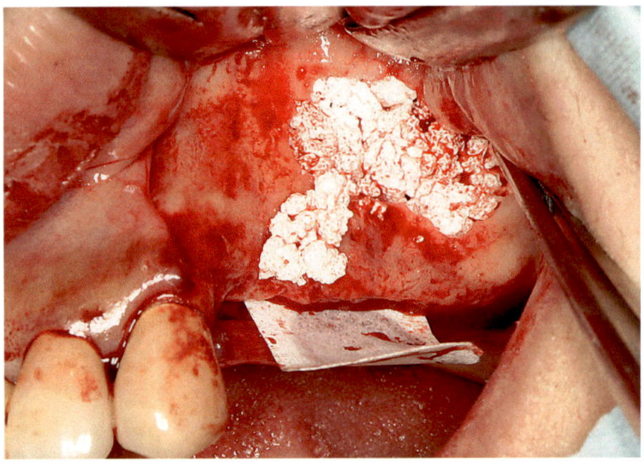

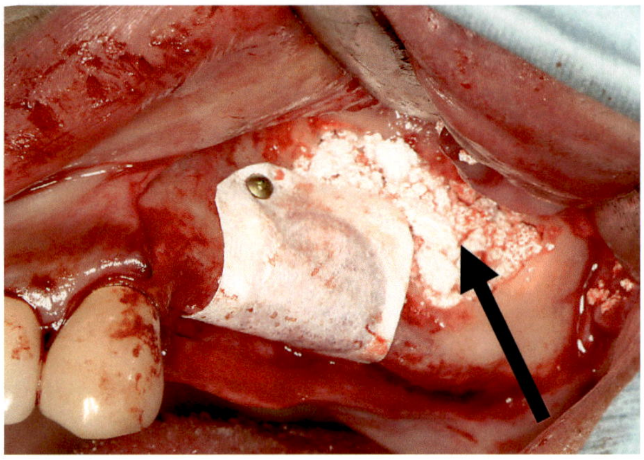

**Figs 4-156 and 4-157** Intraoperative intraoral views.

On the other hand, in the complete coverage group, the granules did not dislocate but remained at the lateral window at 55 sites (94.8%). Type B dislocation was found at one site of the complete coverage group, which was the result of dislocation occurring through a gap created by insufficient fixation of the titanium mesh. Type C dislocation was observed at two sites of the complete coverage group, and arose for different reasons:

- One was due to the pore size of the titanium mesh being larger than that of the granules, allowing movement of the granules through the pores and beyond the adjacent tooth.
- In the other case, the lateral window was covered only by a collagen membrane that was displaced by the large amount of β-TCP granules and led to subsequent dislocation of the granules.

## Risks of release incision (for GBR) over an incompletely covered lateral window

As already mentioned, swelling of the maxillary sinus membrane occurring 1 week after sinus floor elevation increases the internal pressure, leading to buccal dislocation of β-TCP granules through the lateral window. The granules appear to pass through the gap produced between the mucoperiosteal flap and the lateral window. In cases with a recess on the anterior wall of the maxillary sinus, a gap tends to be produced immediately beneath the mucoperiosteal flap, leading to granule dislocations. Further, in cases with simultaneous GBR, the release incision reduces the mechanical strength of the mucoperiosteal flap, and results in increased dislocation of β-TCP granules.

### Clinical report 1: Revelation of sinus floor elevation gained by CT

This patient (a non-smoker) was in the type 2/C incomplete coverage group. The patient with partial edentulism from region 24 to 27 was treated with sinus floor elevation and simultaneous GBR (Figs 4-156 and 4-157). The granules were placed at region 25 and covered with a barrier membrane. However, the barrier membrane did not cover the entire lateral window (black arrow on Fig 4-157). Because simultaneous GBR was performed, the wound was closed after a sufficient release incision.

During the postoperative follow-up, a simple comparison of CT images immediately after and 1 year after the surgery appeared to indicate resorption of granules, but this was deceptive.

Figures 4-158 to 4-163 are the preoperative to 1-year postoperative images. The image taken immediately after the surgery clearly shows that the space created by sinus floor elevation was filled with a sufficient amount of granules (Fig 4-159). One week after the surgery, swelling of the maxillary sinus membrane was found (blue arrows on Fig 4-160; type 2) and some of the granules disappeared (red arrow).

Three months after the surgery, there was no longer any swelling but there was some reduction in the volume gain from sinus floor elevation when compared with the volume immediately following surgery (green arrows on Fig 4-161). One year after the surgery, slight volume reduction was found when compared with the volume 3 months after the surgery, but a radiopaque line of the newly formed maxillary sinus floor was observed (pink arrows on Fig 4-163). The volume at the elevated sinus floor on the sagittal CT 1 year after surgery shows a significant reduction when compared with the volume seen immediately after surgery. However, the most significant reduction is seen at 1 week after surgery.

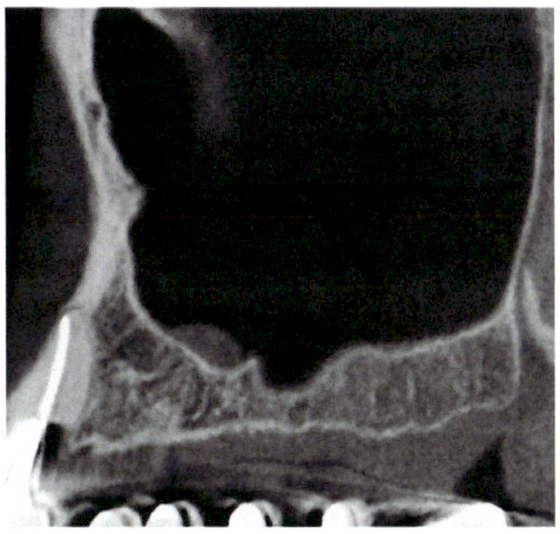

**Fig 4-158** Sagittal CT image immediately before surgery.

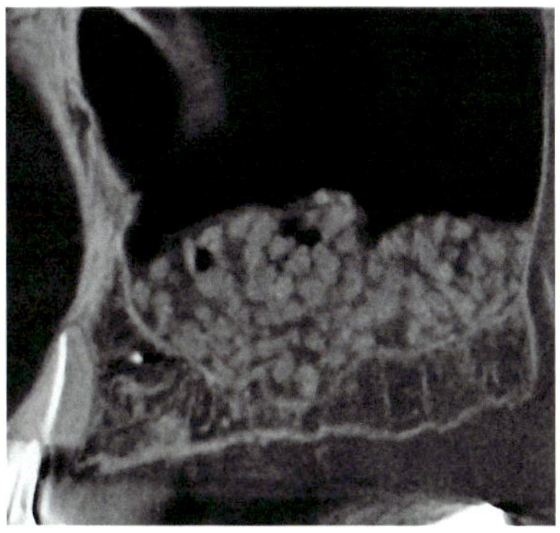

**Fig 4-159** Sagittal CT image immediately after surgery.

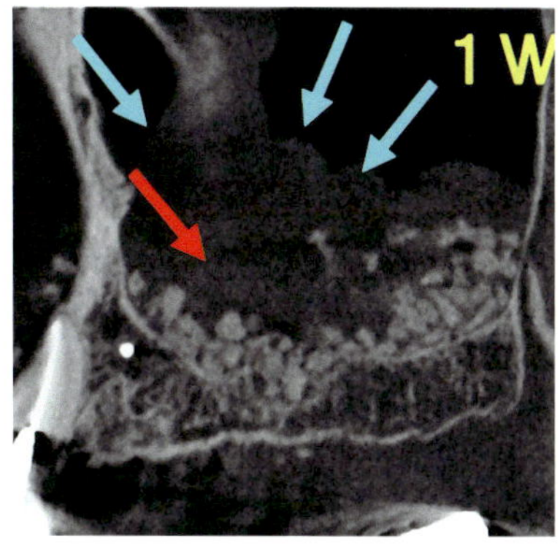


**Fig 4-160** Sagittal CT image 1 week after surgery.

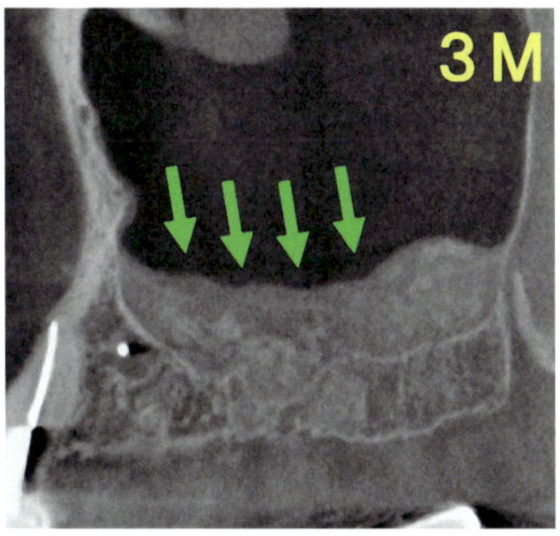


**Fig 4-161** Sagittal CT image 3 months after surgery.

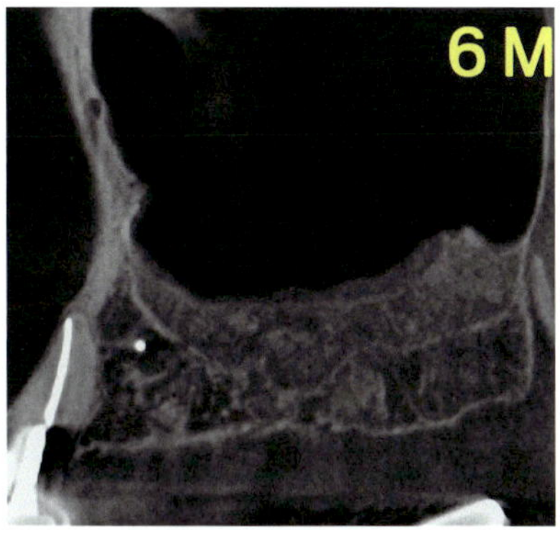


**Fig 4-162** Sagittal CT image 6 months after surgery.

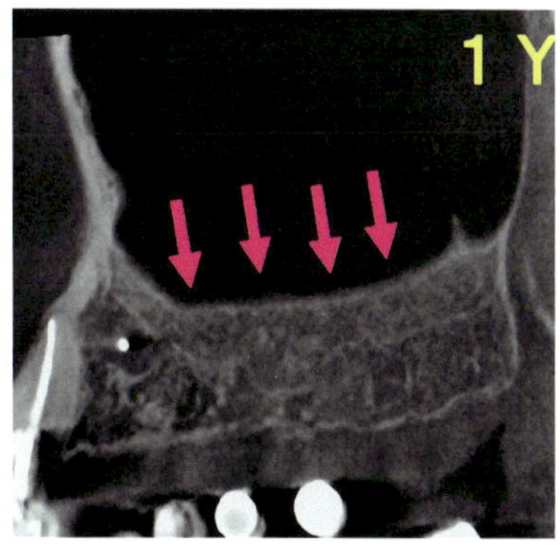


**Fig 4-163** Sagittal CT image 12 months after surgery.

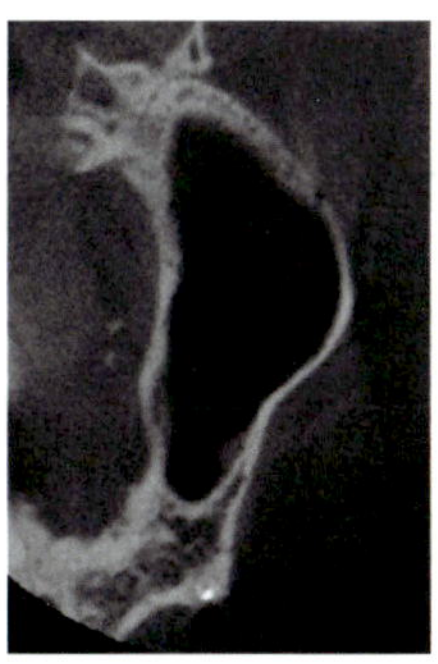

**Fig 4-164** Horizontal CT image immediately before surgery.

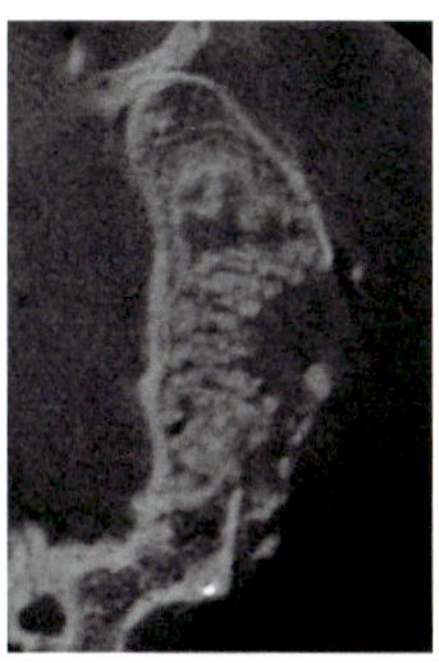

**Fig 4-165** Horizontal CT image immediately after surgery.

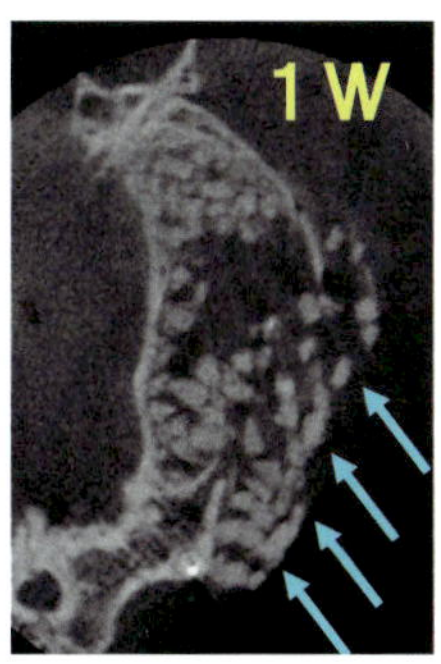


**Fig 4-166** Horizontal CT image 1 week after surgery.

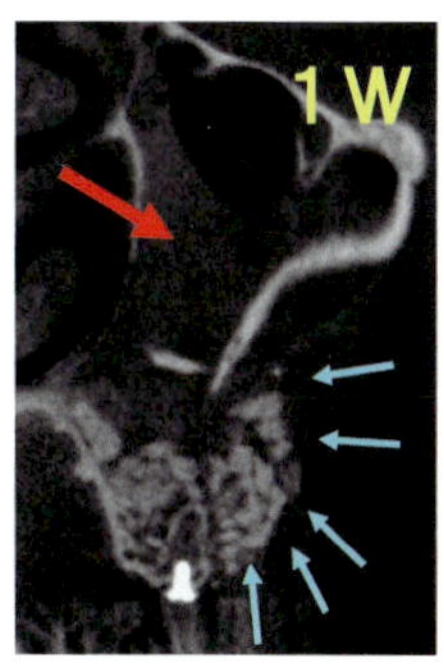


**Fig 4-167** Buccolingual CT image 1 week after surgery.

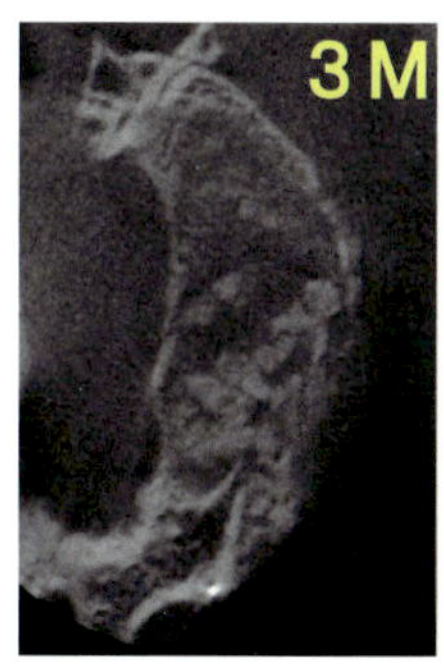


**Fig 4-168** Horizontal CT image 3 months after surgery.

Figures 4-164 to 4-170 are horizontal and buccolingual CT scans. The horizontal CT scan 1 week after surgery shows the dislocation of β-TCP granules to the buccal aspect through the lateral window (blue arrows on Fig 4-166). The buccolingual CT scan, also at 1 week after surgery, indicates a significant swelling of the maxillary sinus membrane (red arrow on Fig 4-167) and the dislocation of granules (blue arrows). The granules that had shifted towards the buccal aspect are observed to have been resorbed on the horizontal CT scan taken at 3 and 12 months and had nearly disappeared (green arrows on Fig 4-170).

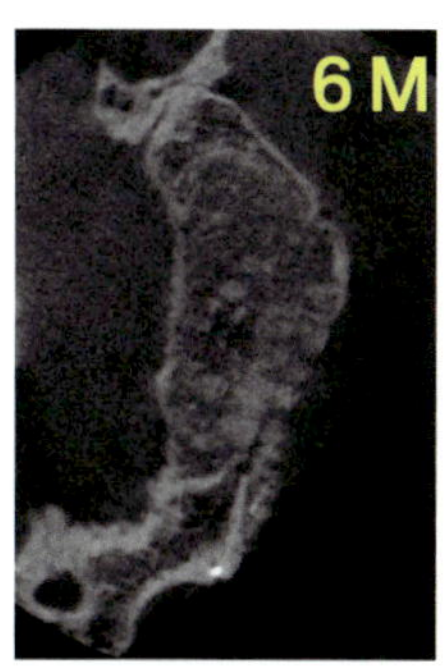


**Fig 4-169** Horizontal CT image 6 months after surgery.

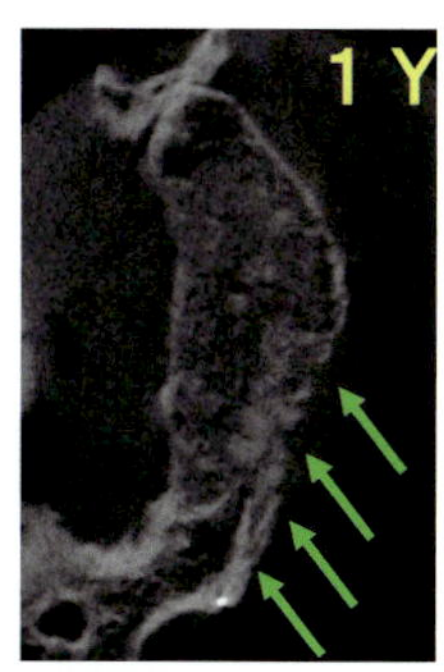


**Fig 4-170** Horizontal CT image 12 months after surgery.

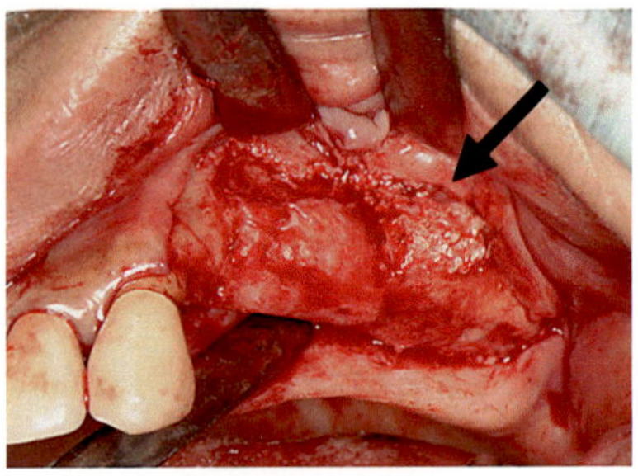

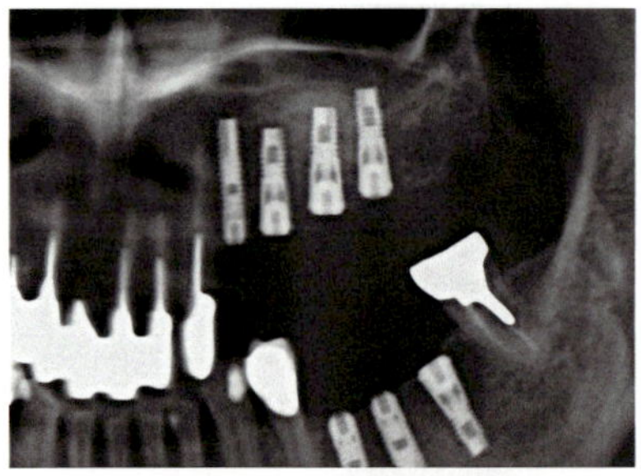

**Fig 4-171** (left) Residual granules at implant placement.

**Fig 4-172** (right) Panoramic view after implant placement.

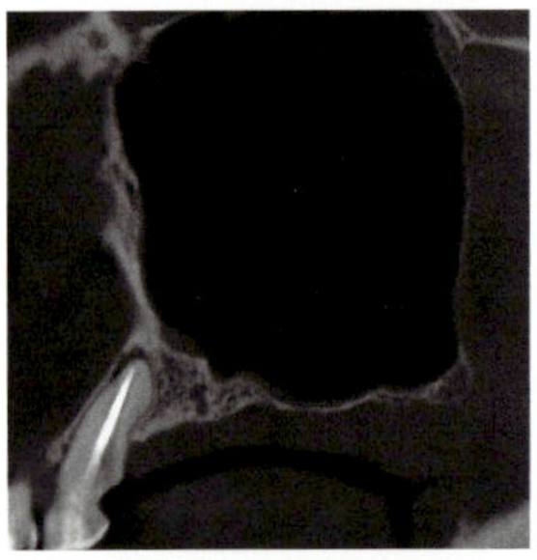

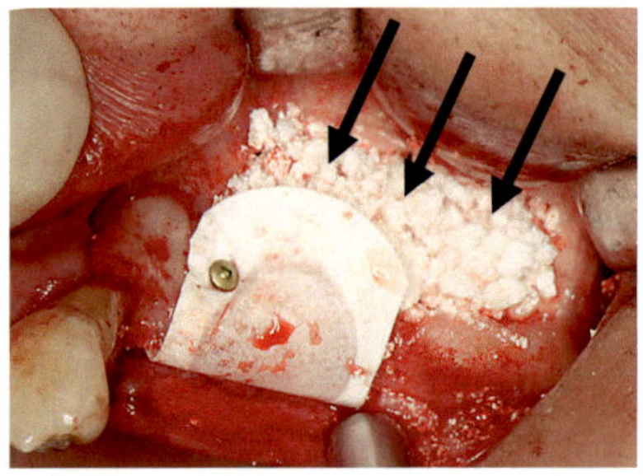

**Fig 4-173** (left) Preoperative CT image.

**Fig 4-174** (right) Intraoperative intraoral view.

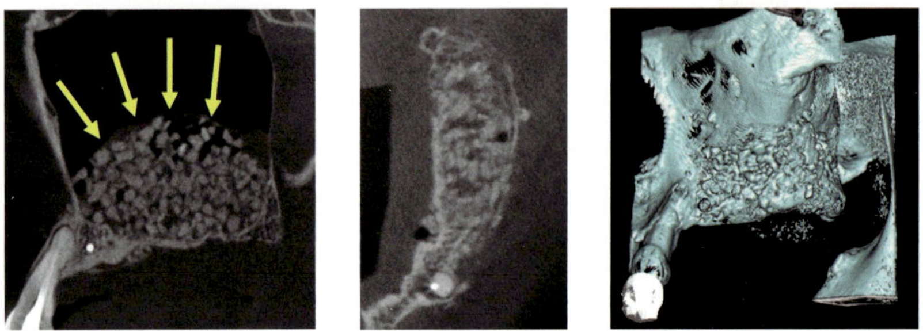

**Figs 4-175 to 4-177** CT images immediately after surgery.

During implant placement 1 year following the surgery, residual β-TCP granules were found at the lateral window (black arrow on Fig 4-171). A panoramic radiograph is also shown (Fig 4-172).

As seen in this case, simple comparison of CT images taken immediately after and 1 year after surgery leads to a misunderstanding that a marked resorption of the β-TCP has occurred.

**! Key Point**

Swelling of the maxillary sinus membrane 1 week after sinus floor elevation and the resulting dislocation of β-TCP granules through the lateral window, and thus the reduction of the granules in the created space, are largely responsible for the reduction in bone gain.

## Clinical report 2: Revelation of sinus floor elevation gained by CT

This patient (a non-smoker) was in the type 3/C incomplete coverage group. The patient with partial edentulism from region 24 to 27 was treated with sinus floor elevation and simultaneous GBR at regions 24 and 25.

Figure 4-173 shows the preoperative situation. Similarly to the case in report 1 above, β-TCP granules were placed and covered with a barrier membrane. However, the barrier membrane did not cover the entire lateral window (black arrows on Fig 4-174). Because simultaneous GBR was undertaken, the wound was closed after an appropriate release incision was made. The CT image immediately after the surgery clearly shows that the space created by sinus floor elevation was filled with a sufficient amount of granules (yellow arrows on Fig 4-175, and Figs 4-176 and 4-177).

**! Key Point**

Sinus floor elevation with simultaneous GBR requires the insertion of a release incision. If the lateral window is not covered completely, there is a risk of β-TCP dislocation through the lateral window.

Figures 4-178 to 4-182 are the CT scans obtained 1 week after the surgery. Significant swelling of the

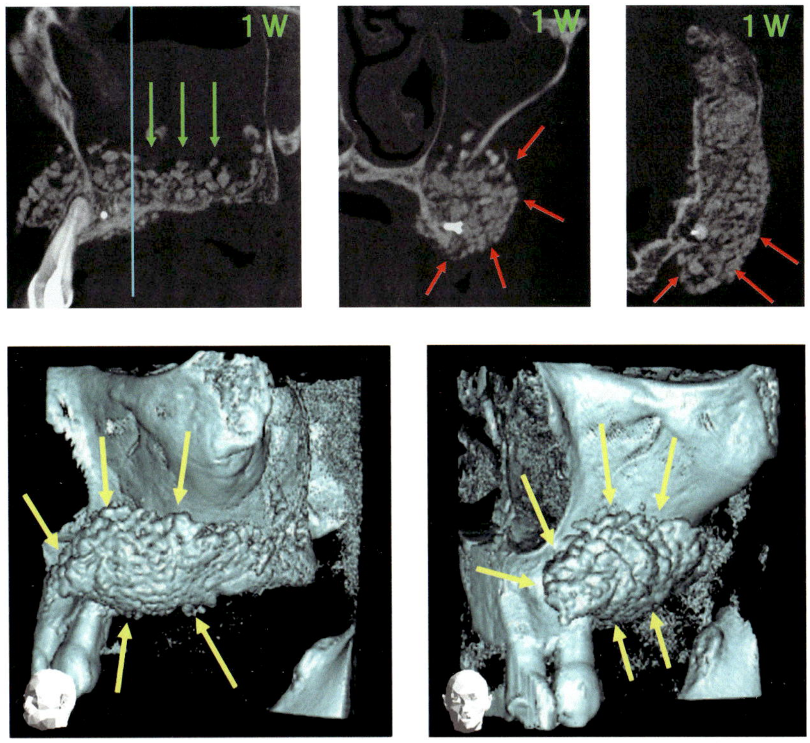


**Figs 4-178 to 4-182** CT images 1 week after surgery.

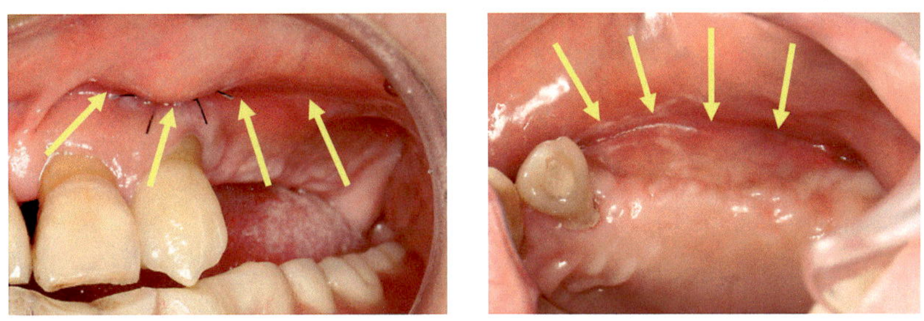

**Figs 4-183 and 4-184** Intraoral views 1 week after surgery.

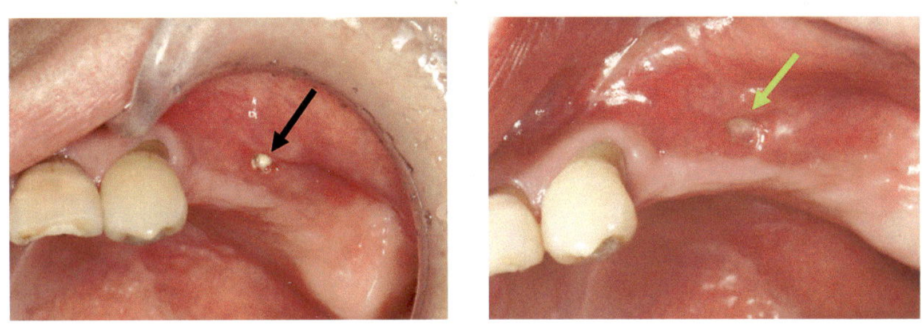

**Figs 4-185 and 4-186** Intraoral views at 6 months after surgery.

maxillary sinus membrane is seen. Further, a large number of granules had shifted towards the buccal aspect through the lateral window (red arrows on Figs 4-179 and 4-180). The dislocated granules were beyond the adjacent tooth (yellow arrows on Figs 4-181 and 4-182), and the amount of β-TCP in the augmented area was strikingly reduced (green arrows on Fig 4-178).

Figures 4-183 and 4-184 are the intraoral views. There is swelling at the buccogingival transition zone from region 22 to 26 (yellow arrows). Something hard, which was considered to be the dislocated β-TCP, was felt immediately beneath the swollen mucosa.

> **! Key Point**
>
> The maxillary sinus membrane swelling occurring 1 week after surgery poses the risk of infection.

There was postoperative follow-up and additional treatment (Figs 4-185 to 4-190). The bulging of the gingiva from region 22 to 26 gradually decreased. Six months after the surgery, however, exposure of β-TCP granules occurred on the buccal gingiva at region 25 (black arrow on Fig 4-185). Barrier membrane was found immediately under the β-TCP granules surgically removed (green arrow on Fig 4-186).

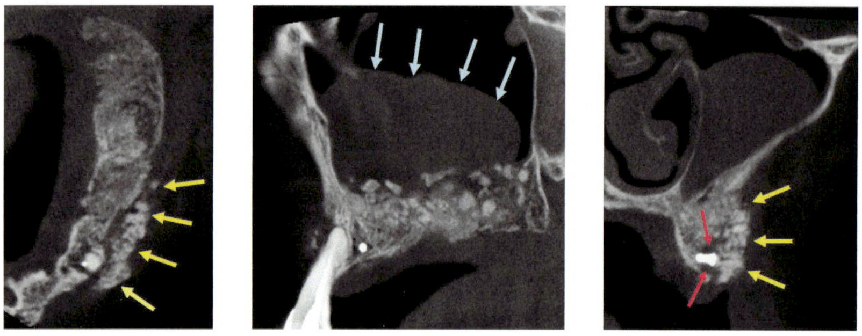

**Figs 4-187 to 4-189** CT views at 6 months after surgery.

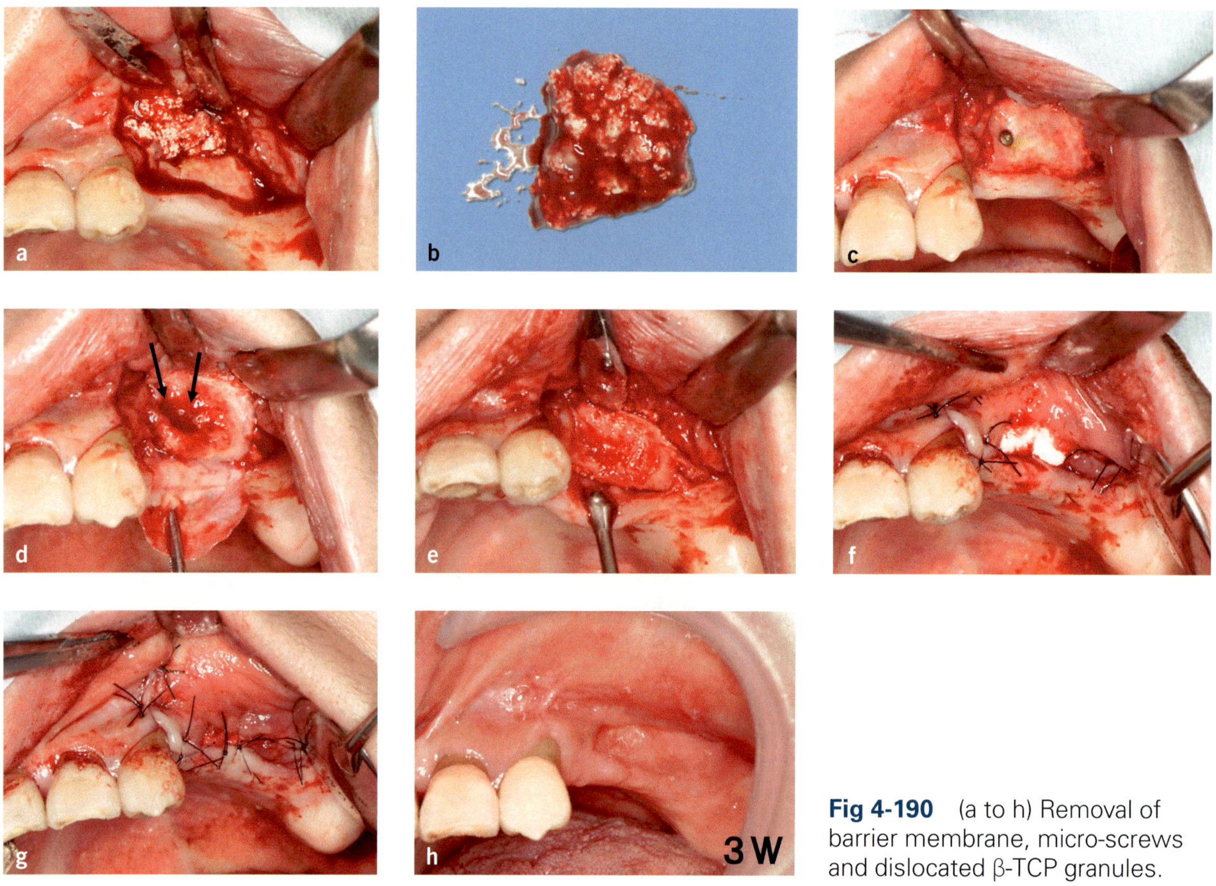


**Fig 4-190** (a to h) Removal of barrier membrane, micro-screws and dislocated β-TCP granules.

A CT scan revealed that the majority of the dislocated granules had been resorbed but the granules on the barrier membrane remained unresorbed (yellow arrows on Figs 4-187 and 4-189). Swelling of the maxillary sinus membrane persisted, which indicated inflammation of the augmented sinus area. Further, alveolar bone resorption was found around the micro-screw (pink arrows on Fig 4-189), thus revealing inflammation of the GBR area.

The barrier membrane, micro-screw and dislocated granules were removed to prevent the risk of infection spreading as a result of the exposed barrier membrane (Fig 4-190). When the flap was reflected, dislocated granules were found in the region from 23 to 25 and were taken out. Removing the micro-screw and barrier membrane revealed a crater-like bone resorption around the micro-screw (black arrows on Fig 4-190d).

Although no purulent discharge was observed during removal surgery, there was a sign of infection in the area treated with sinus floor elevation and GBR. The soft tissue immediately beneath the barrier membrane was removed by curettage, a cross-linked collagen membrane (Terudermis; Olympus Terumo Materials) was then placed over the mucosal defect, and the wound was closed (Figs 4-190e–g). Three weeks later, the mucosal defect had covered over with epithelium, indicative of favorable wound healing (Fig 4-190h).

On the CT images obtained 1 year later, a radiopaque line indicating the newly formed maxillary sinus floor was observed, although the maxillary sinus

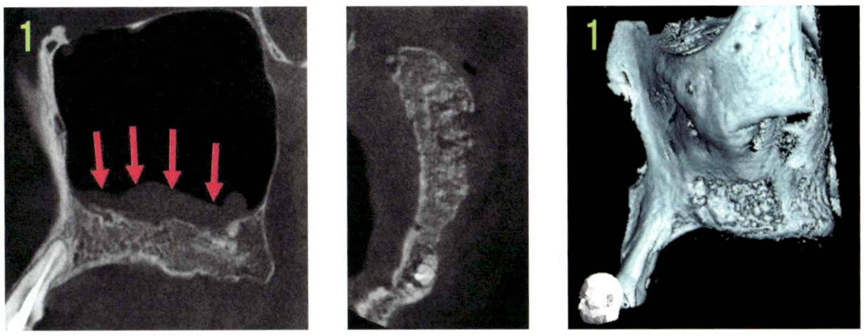


**Figs 4-191 to 4-193** CT images 1 year after sinus floor elevation.

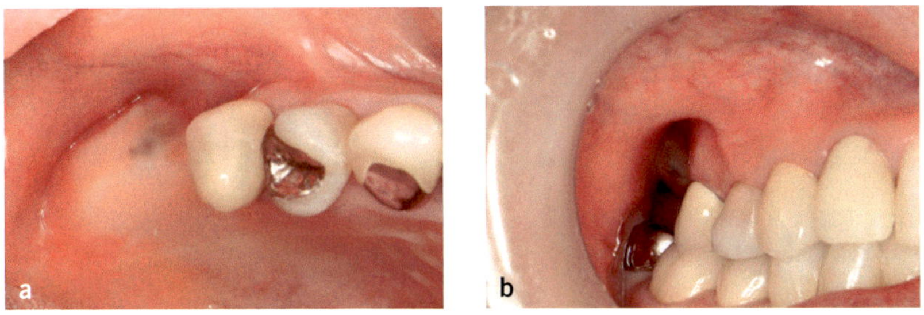

**Fig 4-194** (a and b) Preoperative intraoral views.

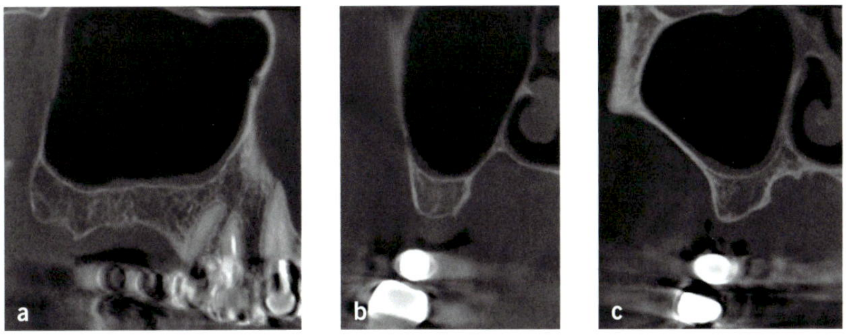

**Fig 4-195** (a to c) Preoperative CT views.

membrane still showed some swelling (pink arrows on Fig 4-191). When compared with the CT image immediately after surgery, however, there was a marked decrease in the volume of the augmented mass and the placement of an implant of sufficient length was deemed impossible.

This case demonstrated that the maxillary sinus membrane swelling occurring 1 week after surgery not only reduces the volume of augmented mass but also poses the risk of postoperative infection.

## Drawback of titanium mesh with pore size larger than a β-TCP granule

Coverage of a lateral window with a titanium mesh to prevent the β-TCP granules from being pushed out of the lateral window by the pressure of membrane swelling was described in an earlier section. However, the author experienced a case in which a titanium mesh with a pore size larger than a β-TCP granule was used. As seen in the case described below, the pressure generated by the membrane swelling is stronger than might be expected, and buccal shift of granules through the titanium mesh could not be prevented.

## Clinical report 3: Granule dislocation through a titanium mesh

> **! Key Point**
>
> The pressure produced by the maxillary sinus membrane swelling is so strong that it exerts an "explosion-like" influence in every direction.

This patient was in the type 3/C complete coverage group. The patient with loss of teeth 16 and 17 was treated with sinus floor elevation and simultaneous implant placement (Figs 4-194 to 4-196).

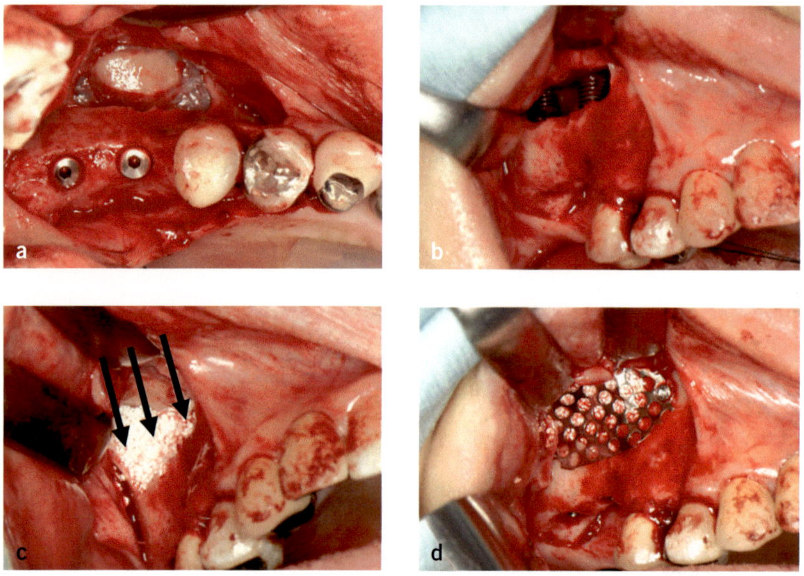


**Fig 4-196** (a to d) Intraoperative intraoral views.

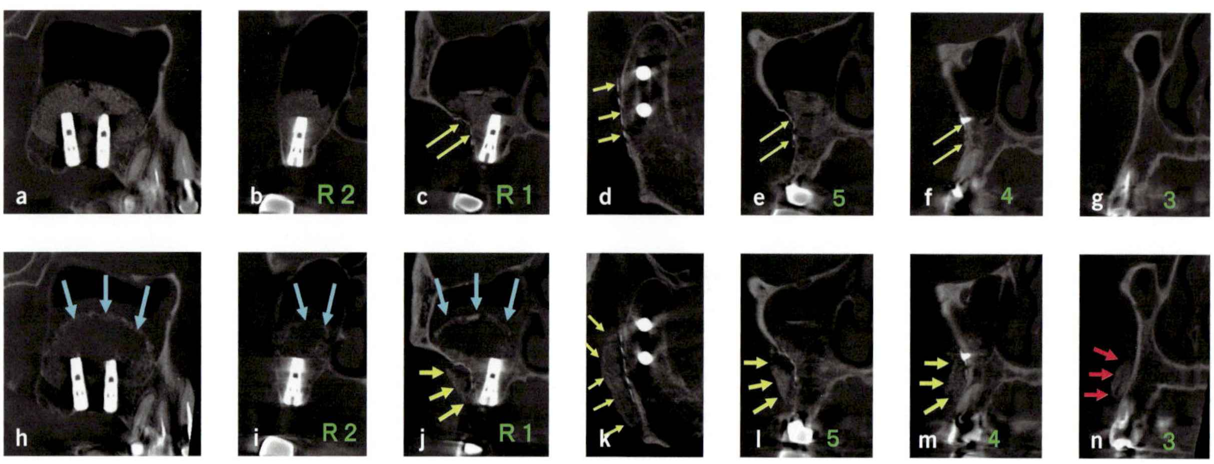


**Fig 4-197** (a to n) Postoperative follow-up on a weekly basis. *Top row:* immediately after surgery; *bottom row:* 1 week after surgery.

Because good primary stability was achieved for both implants (Fig 4-196a), β-TCP granules were placed into the gap around the implant (Figs 4-196b and c) and the lateral window was covered with a titanium mesh. Looking back at the intraoperative photos, it is clear that the pore size of the mesh is larger than a β-TCP granule (Fig 4-196d). For this patient, no release incision in the periostium was made but the anterior wall of the maxillary sinus presented a concave shape.

CT images were obtained immediately following the surgery (top row in Fig 4-197). Granules around the implants and the titanium mesh over the lateral window are clearly visible (yellow arrows on Figs 4-197c to f).

CT images obtained 1 week later (bottom row in Fig 4-197) show swelling of the maxillary sinus membrane. The upper area of the filling granules was pushed upwards in a dome shape (blue arrows on Figs 4-197h–j). Buccal shift of granules through the pores of the titanium mesh can be seen (yellow arrows on Figs 4-197j–m), and the dislocation extended to the buccal aspect of tooth 13 (red arrow on Fig 4-197n).

Based on the observation that the β-TCP granules in this area were pushed upward, it seems that the pressure produced by the swelling of the sinus membrane applies not only a unidirectional effect but exerts an "explosion-like" impact in every direction. Intraoral views 10 days after the surgery show swelling in the buccogingival transition zone from region 13 to region 16 (green arrows on Fig 4-198). The presence of hard material, probably the β-TCP granules, was detected immediately under the mucosa.

Figures 4-199a–g are the CT images obtained 3 months after the surgery. Swelling of the maxillary sinus membrane is no longer seen and the β-TCP granules, which had been pushed up, had settled

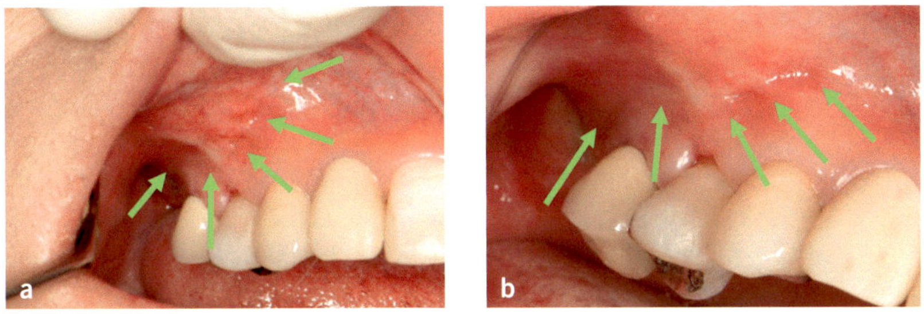


**Fig 4-198** (a and b) Intraoral views 10 days after surgery.

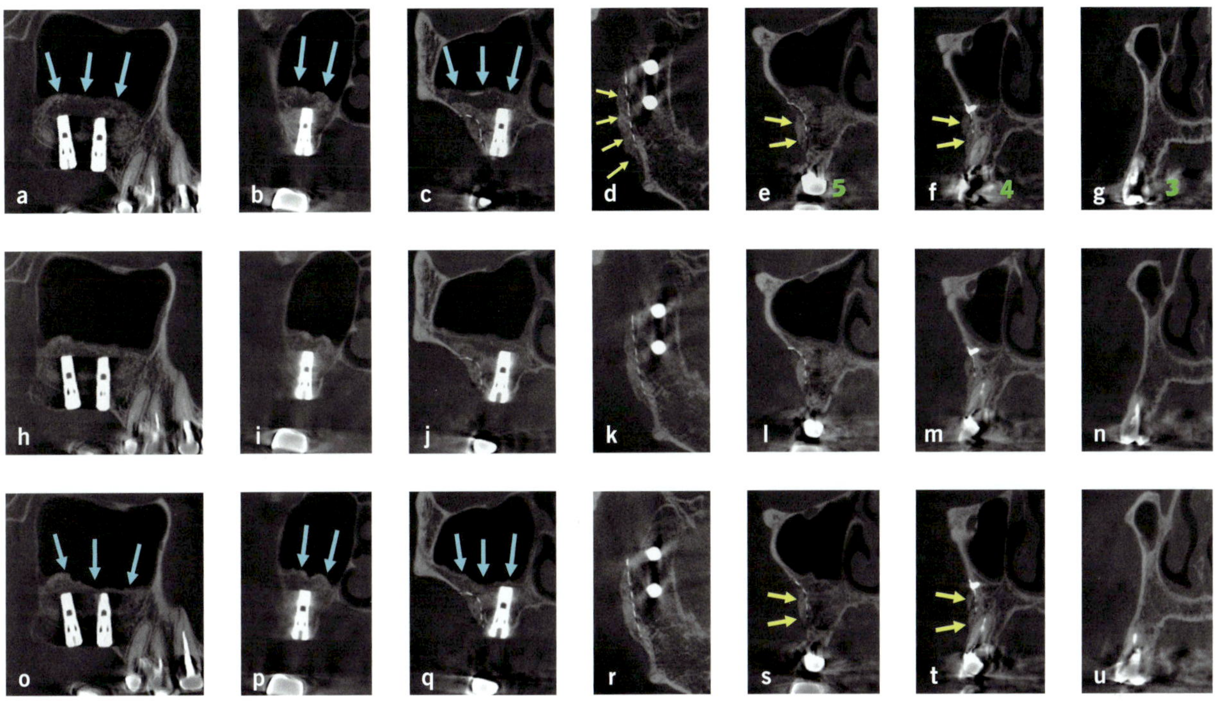


**Fig 4-199** (a to u) Postoperative follow-up on a monthly basis. *Top row*: 3 months after surgery; middle row: 6 months after surgery; *bottom row*: 9 months after surgery.

down (blue arrows on Figs 4-199a to c). The granules that had shifted on the buccal aspect manifested a resorption tendency (yellow arrows on Figs 4-199d to f), and the granules at region 13 had disappeared (Fig 4-199g).

Figures 4-199h to n are the corresponding CT images obtained 6 months after the surgery. No swelling was found at the maxillary sinus membrane and the contours of individual β-TCP granules had becoming less distinct.

Figures 4-199o to u are the corresponding CT images obtained 9 months after the surgery. A radiopaque line indicating the newly formed maxillary sinus floor is observed, and β-TCP granules are fusing with each other. Dislocated granules are still present on the buccal aspect in the area from R1 to tooth 14 (yellow arrows on Figs 4-199q to t), but at a slightly decreased level when compared with that seen 3 months after surgery.

Second surgery was performed 12 months after the first operation (Fig 4-200). Granules were still present on the buccal surface of the titanium mesh (yellow arrows on Fig 4-200a), but these granules did not have any mechanical strength and the titanium mesh was removed without difficulty. Hard tissue incorporating granules was present in the lateral window area, but the mechanical strength of this hard tissue was similar to that of foamed styrene (blue arrows on Fig 4-200d). No mobility of the implant was detected during healing abutment connection; thus the implant had successfully osseointegrated.

Figure 4-201 shows CT images obtained 1, 1.5, 2, and 3 years after the sinus floor elevation. A sufficient area of radiopacity was found around R1 and R2. Two years after this surgery, cortical-bone–like radiopaque lines were observed in the area corresponding to the lateral window and the newly formed maxillary sinus floor (blue arrows on Figs 4-201c and g). Further, cancel-

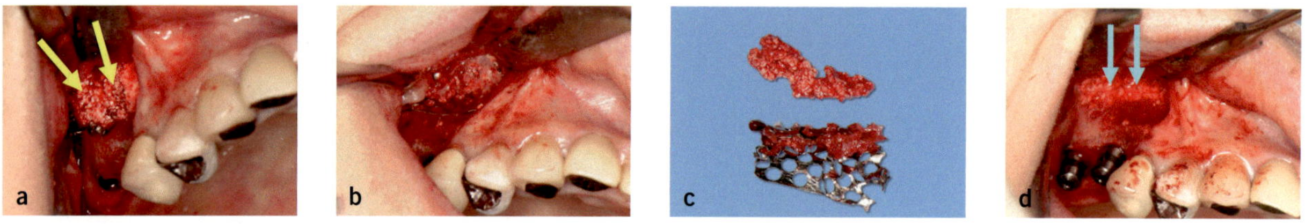


**Fig 4-200** (a to d) Intraoperative intraoral views during the second surgery.

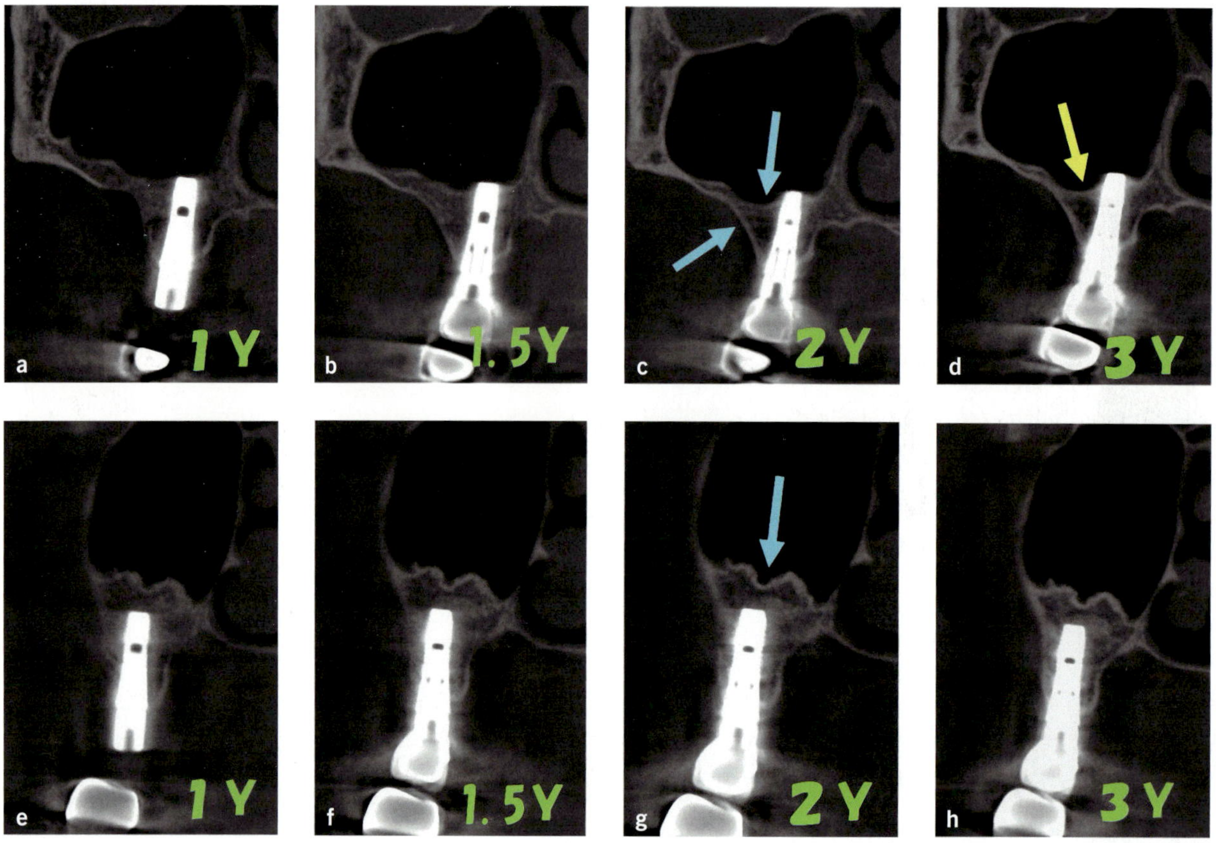


**Fig 4-201** (a to h) CT images obtained 1, 1.5, 2, and 3 years after the sinus floor elevation. Top row: R1; bottom row: R2.

lous-bone–like radiopacity was observed in the center of the augmented bone area, which suggests that active remodeling in the augmented mass had settled down. In the area peripheral to R1, 3 years after this surgery, a slight lowering of the newly formed sinus floor can be observed (yellow arrow on Fig 4-201d), but no swelling of the maxillary sinus membrane was found around the implant apex, indicating the absence of clinical problems.

## Doubtful security of collagen membrane alone

When a maxillary sinus to be treated is large and has complicated inner morphology, osteotomy of a large lateral window is indispensable for adequate elevation of the sinus membrane. If the anterior wall of the maxillary sinus is thin, it is difficult to affix a titanium mesh with micro-screws.

The author experienced a case in which bone substitute granules shifted when collagen membranes, which were stacked in pairs over the lateral window on a thin anterior wall, were pushed away. This demonstrates the power of the pressure produced by the swelling of the maxillary sinus membrane is very strong. When the anterior wall of the maxillary sinus is thin, it may be safe to drill a small hole into the anterior wall and attach the titanium mesh by bone-suturing with a nylon thread or a stainless steel wire.

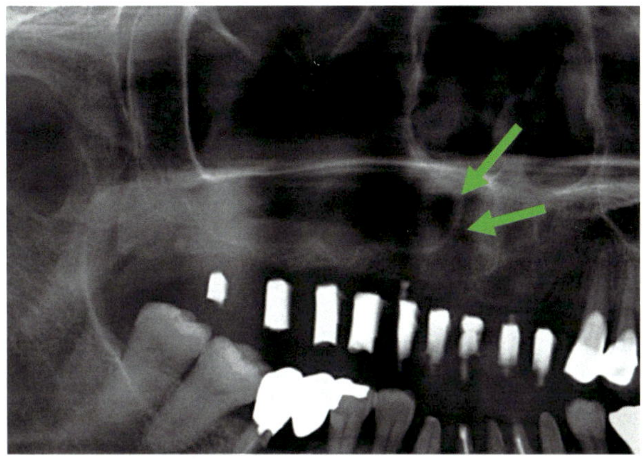

**Fig 4-202** Panoramic view before treatment.

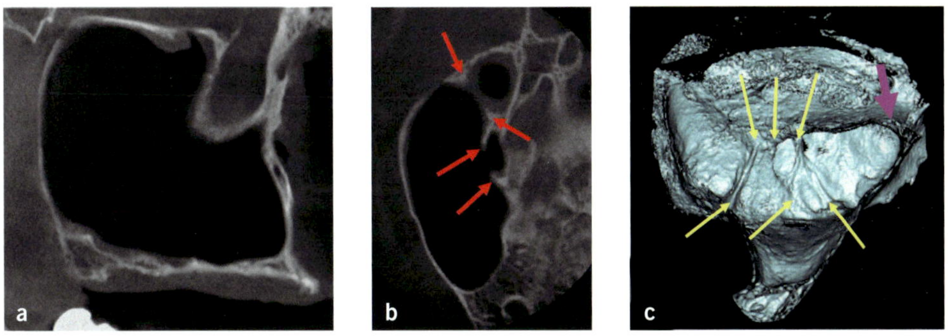


**Fig 4-203** (a to c) CT images before treatment.

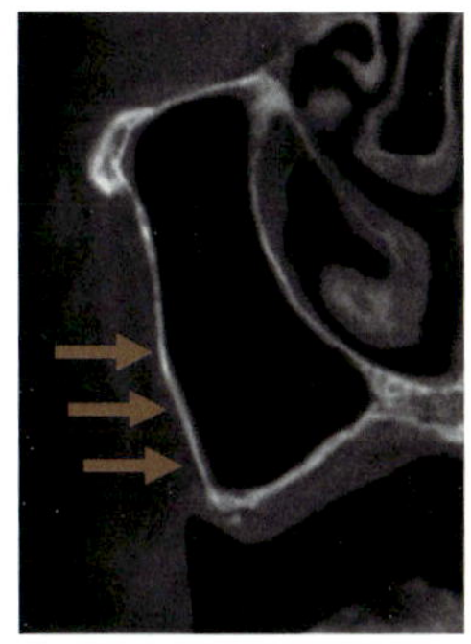

**Fig 4-204** Buccolingual CT image before treatment.

## Clinical report 4: Mishap of lateral window coverage with collagen membrane alone

> **! Key Point**
>
> A maxillary sinus that is large and presents with complicated inner morphology requires osteotomy of a large lateral window.

This patient was in the type 3/C complete coverage group. The patient with loss of teeth 11 to 17, 21, and 22 was referred for implant treatment. Downward and forward growth of the maxillary sinus observed on the panoramic radiograph indicated the need for sinus floor elevation (green arrows on Fig 4-202).

Figure 4-203 shows preoperative CT scans. These revealed complicated morphology of the sinus with the presence of septa at region 17 and medial wall (red arrows on Fig 4-203b). Further, when viewed from above by the volume rendering image, several septa were observed (yellow arrows on Fig 4-203c), and the anterior portion of the sinus cavity reached immediately beneath the nasal cavity (pink arrow on Fig 4-203c).

Creation of a large lateral window was necessary to ensure adequate elevation of the maxillary sinus membrane. A buccolingual CT scan indicated that the bone of the anterior wall was very thin (brown arrows on Fig 4-204), and it became evident that titanium mesh fixation by means of micro-screws would be difficult.

> **! Key Point**
>
> Because the bone of the anterior wall was extremely thin, collagen membrane (Terudermis; Olympus Terumo Biomaterials, Japan), stacked in pairs, was employed instead of affixing a titanium mesh with micro-screws. Moreover, the wound was closed without making a release incision in the periostium.

The lateral window was created according to standard procedure and the maxillary sinus membrane was elevated (Fig 4-205). When the maxillary sinus has a complicated morphology, as was the case for this patient, a scalpel with a small head (Martin) is useful in elevating the maxillary sinus membrane (Fig 4-206).

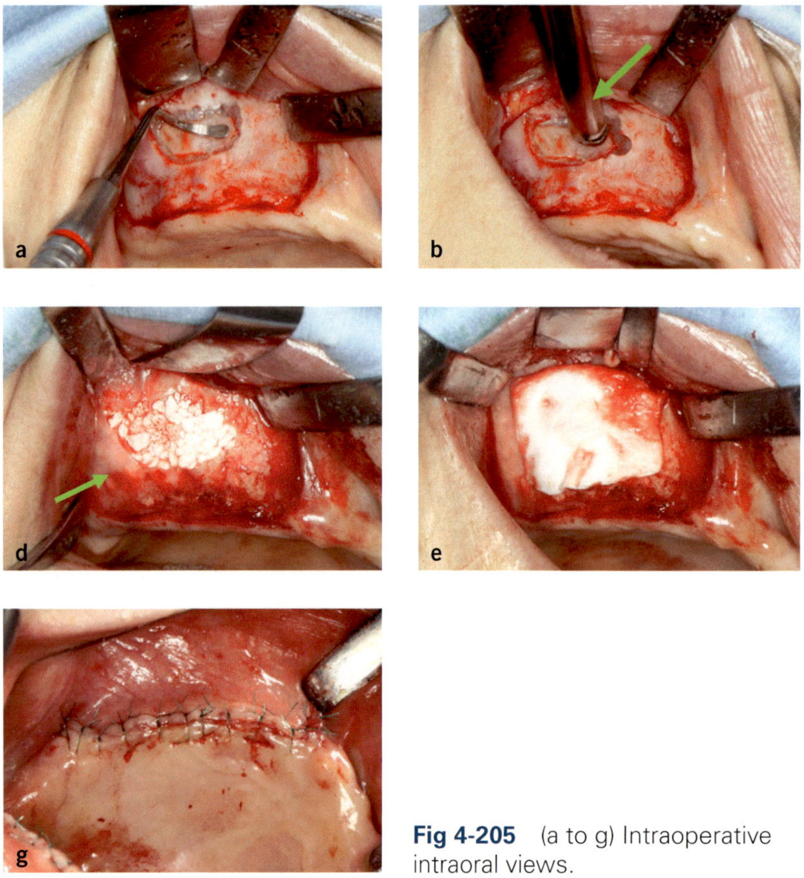

Fig 4-205 (a to g) Intraoperative intraoral views.

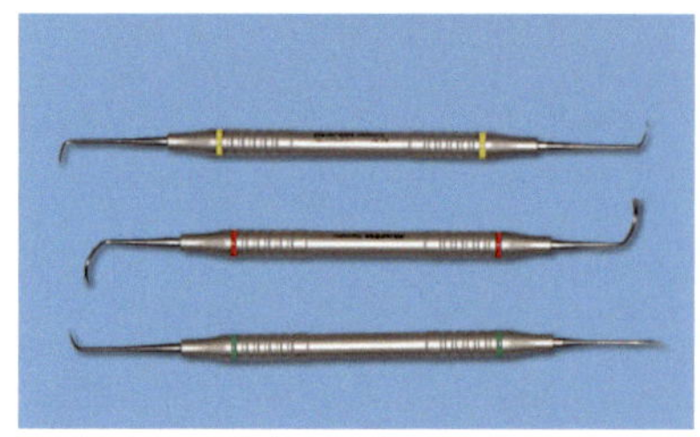

Fig 4-206 Suitable scalpels.

When removing the bone around the lateral window to gain better visibility, Kerrison (Martin) is recommended (green arrow on Fig 4-205b). At the medial wall of the maxillary sinus, the membrane in the posterior and anterior areas was dissected and elevated superiorly without any damage to the membrane. However, a large bone defect was produced at the lateral window (Fig 4-205c). The anterior wall of this patient's maxillary sinus was so thin that the β-TCP granules placed in the space were visible through the bone (green arrow on Fig 4-205d).

The panoramic radiograph and CT images taken immediately after surgery show that the space created by sinus floor elevation was sufficiently filled with β-TCP granules (Figs 4-207a–d).

CT images were obtained 1 week after the surgery (Figs 4-207e–g). The maxillary sinus membrane was swollen and the granules were translocating past the lateral window (yellow arrows). There were no findings of pain or postoperative infection, but swelling at the buccogingival transition zone was observed, and something hard was felt immediately beneath the swollen mucosa (Figs 4-207h and i).

CT images were obtained 1 month after the surgery (Figs 4-207j–l). Swelling of the maxillary sinus membrane was no longer seen. The raised clump of dislocated β-TCP granules had flattened, but some particles remained on the buccal aspect of the lateral window (green arrows on Figs 4-207k and l). Wound healing was good, and a temporary maxillary denture was provided to the patient. No sign of postoperative infection or inflammation was found (Figs 4-207m and n).

Figure 4-208 shows volume rendering CT images for comparison. At 1 week, granules were translocating toward the buccal aspects in every direction (Fig 4-208c). At 1 month, the displaced granules failed to return to their original position but remained on the buccal areas (Fig 4-208d). These observations suggest that the pressure generated by the swelling of the maxillary sinus membrane and subsequent displacement of granules is very strong, and installation of a collagen membrane alone will be inadequate to prevent granule dislocation.

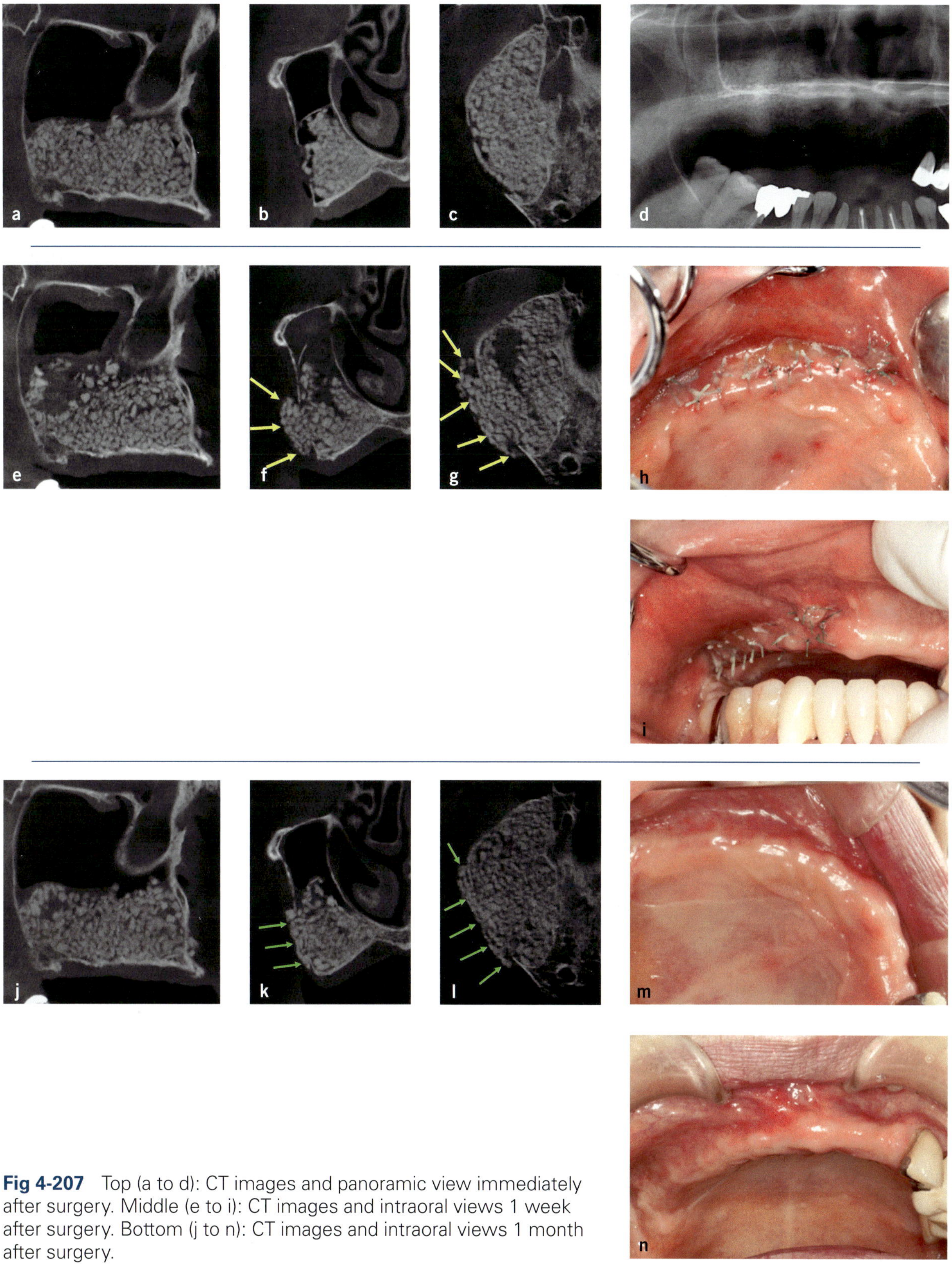

**Fig 4-207** Top (a to d): CT images and panoramic view immediately after surgery. Middle (e to i): CT images and intraoral views 1 week after surgery. Bottom (j to n): CT images and intraoral views 1 month after surgery.

> **! Key Point**
>
> The pressure generated by the swelling of the maxillary sinus membrane and subsequent displacement of β-TCP granules is very strong, and installation of a collagen membrane alone will be inadequate to prevent granule dislocation.

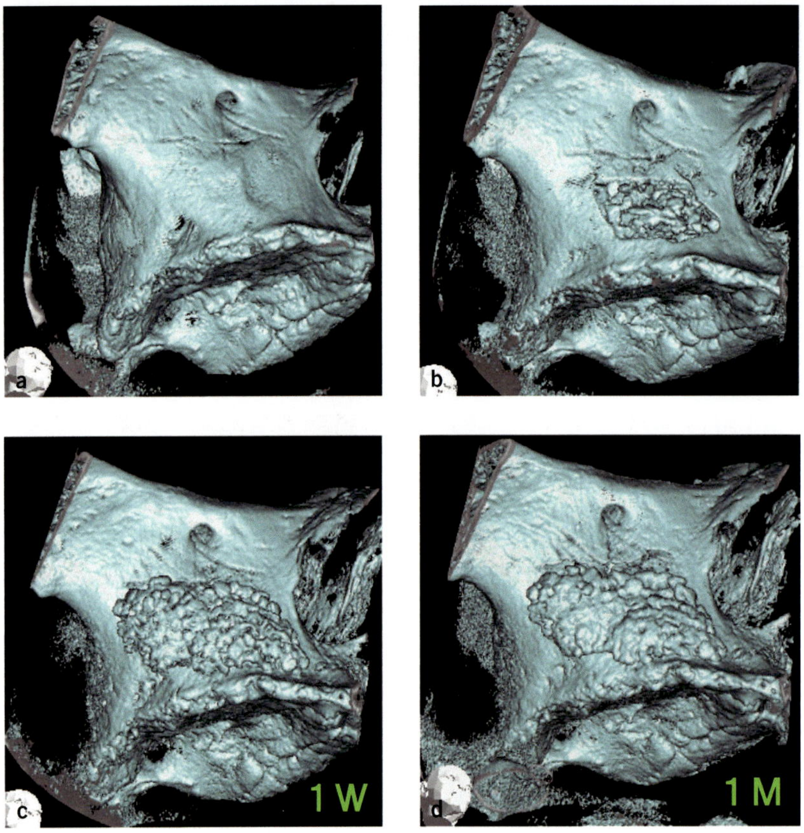


**Fig 4-208** Volume rendering CT images: (a) before, (b) immediately after, and (c) 1 week and (d) 1 month after surgery.

## Firmness of closure of the lateral window

For the sinus floor elevation procedure, firmly closing the lateral window with a titanium mesh and micro-screws will help prevent dislocation of bone substitutes that results from swelling of the maxillary sinus membrane. In cases with a recess on the anterior wall of the maxillary sinus or involving the inclusion of a release incision, a dead space is created between the mucoperiosteal flap and the lateral window through which bone substitutes may dislocate.

It is impossible to predict the severity of postoperative swelling of the maxillary sinus membrane. Therefore, firm closure of the lateral window will be important to increase the predictability of sinus floor elevation outcomes.

### Clinical report 5: Clinical course of lateral window closure

**! Key Point**

The author always closes the lateral window with titanium mesh to prevent dislocation of β-TCP granules resulting from swelling of the maxillary sinus membrane.

This patient (a non-smoker) was in the type 3/A group. The patient visited our clinic for implant treatment of the partial edentulism from tooth 14 to tooth 17. Owing to the downward growth of the maxillary sinus, the patient was treated with sinus floor elevation (Fig 4-209).

After sufficient elevation of the maxillary sinus membrane and placement of β-TCP granules, the lateral window was closed with a titanium mesh that was affixed with self-tapping micro-screws (ProSeed, Japan). The granules, titanium mesh and micro-screws are visible on the panoramic radiograph obtained immediately after surgery (Fig 4-210).

Figure 4-211 shows a series of CT images taken immediately after surgery to 1 year. A dead space was identified on the buccal side of the titanium mesh on the buccolingual CT scan immediately after surgery (green arrow on Fig 4-211b). In the case of this patient, no release incision of the periostium was made. However, in cases with a recess on the anterior wall of the maxillary sinus, a dead space tends to occur on the buccal side of the lateral window after wound closure. CT images obtained 1 week after surgery (Figs 4-211c and d) showed substantial swelling of the maxillary sinus membrane, but no dislocation of β-TCP granules was found on the buccal aspect of the lateral window (blue arrow). The bone plate of the lateral window was vertically pushed up with the swelling of the maxillary

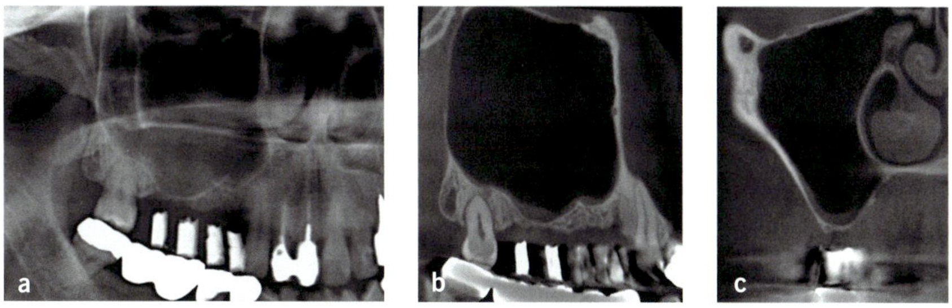

Fig 4-209 (a to c) Panoramic and CT images before surgery.

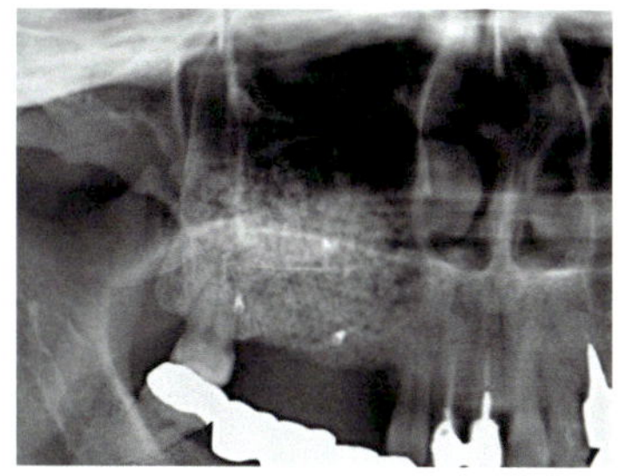

Fig 4-210 Panoramic view immediately after surgery.

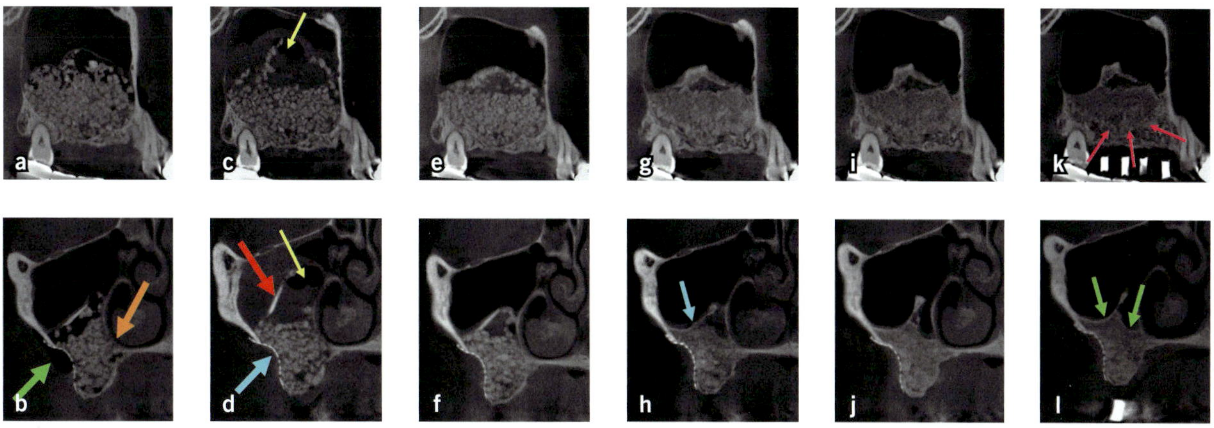

Fig 4-211 CT images: (a and b) immediately after surgery; (c and d) at 1 week; (e and f) at 3 months; (g and h) at 6 months; (I and j) at 9 months; (k and l) at 12 months.

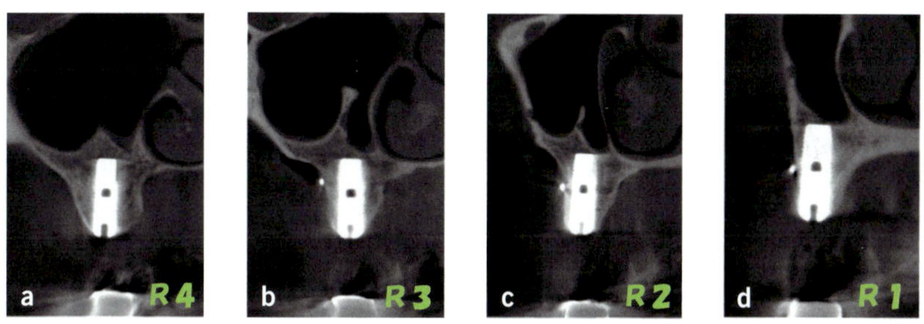


Fig 4-212 (a to d) CT images of the four implants.

sinus membrane (red arrow). The air around the granules, which was observed on the CT image immediately after surgery, formed a pneumatic space in the upper part of the augmented area (yellow arrow).

On the CT images 3 months after surgery, both the membrane swelling and pneumatic space disappeared, but no change was observed in the volume of the granules. A radiopaque line (blue arrow on Fig 4-211h) of the newly formed sinus floor was observed on the CT image 6 months after surgery, and the size of each individual β-TCP granule in the marginal region of the augmented sinus area became smaller. On the other hand, a reduction of bone level was observed in the medial area of the maxillary sinus (currently under investigation). The volume decrease is more frequent in cases where depression towards the nasal cavity is observed in the medial part of the maxillary sinus on the CT scan before surgery. Such was the case for this patient (orange arrow on Fig 4-211b). Further decrease of the size of each individual β-TCP granule was shown on the CT image 9 months after surgery (Figs 4-211i and j).

On the CT images 1 year after surgery, the radiopaque line of the newly formed sinus floor was more defined than before (green arrows on Fig 4-211l), but residual granules were found at the center of the augmented area (red arrows on Fig 4-211k).

The titanium mesh was removed 1 year after surgery and the implants were placed (Figs 4-212 to 4-214). A hard bone-like tissue, in which residual β-TCP granules were incorporated, was observed in the area of the lateral window. Four implants with diameter 4 mm and length 13 mm were inserted and these implants achieved good primary stability.

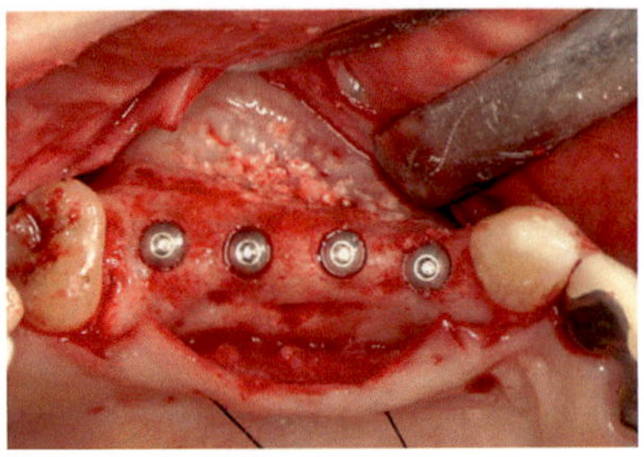

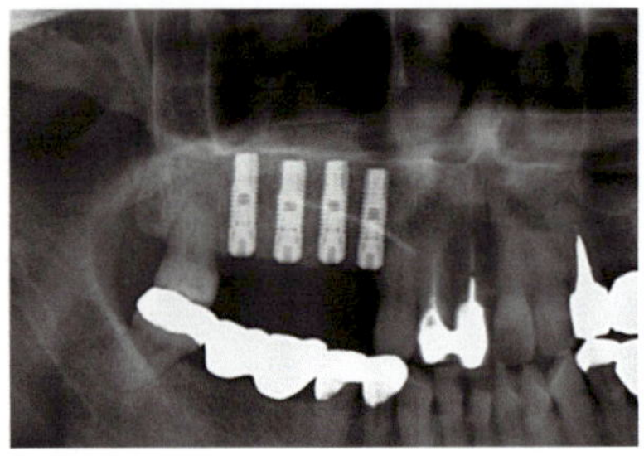

**Fig 4-213** (left) Intraoral view of the implants.

**Fig 4-214** (right) Panoramic view of the implants.

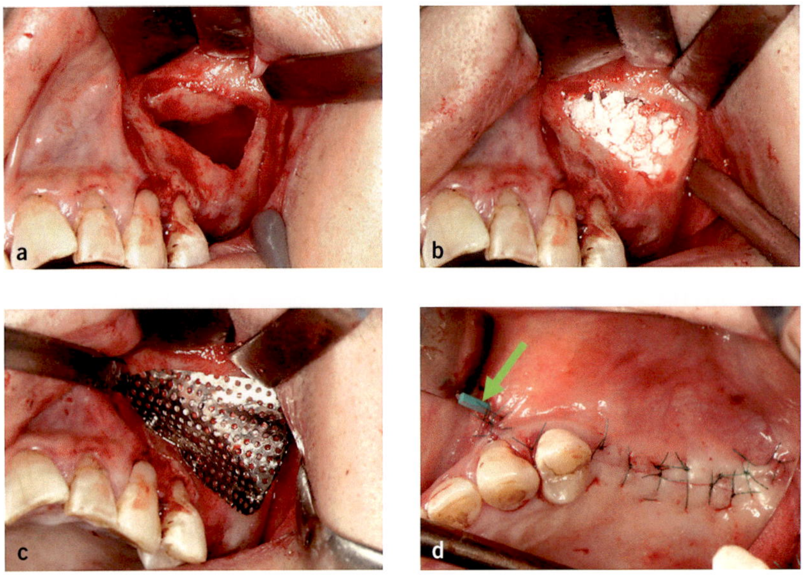


**Fig 4-215** (a to d) Intraoperative intraoral views.

## Alleviation of facial swelling by drain insertion

Although variable among patients, sinus floor elevation is often associated with significant facial swelling. Postoperative swelling is greatest on day 2, and often extends from the cheek to the eyelid. Administration of steroids is regarded as an effective means to alleviate postoperative swelling. The author administered steroids to three patients after sinus floor elevation, but the postoperative swelling of the maxillary sinus membrane and the face was unresponsive to the drugs. The author, henceforth, generally refrains from prescribing steroids to patients.

Once a titanium mesh is used to close the lateral window, a drain can be inserted through a vertical incision. This can remove resulting surgical wound exudate, thus lessening the extent of postoperative facial swelling.

### Clinical report 6: Drain insertion when the lateral window is closed with titanium mesh

This patient underwent sinus floor elevation on the left side. After placing β-TCP granules, a titanium mesh was placed over the lateral window and fixed with micro-screws (Fig 4-215). A drain was inserted through the vertical incision, and the drain and mucosa were sutured together for fixation (green arrow on Fig 4-215d). The drain used was a Penrose (Fuji Systems , Japan) with a green radiopaque line to facilitate placement verification. On the panoramic radiograph immediately after surgery, the radiopaque granules, titanium mesh, micro-screws and drain can be seen (yellow arrow on Fig 4-216). Figure 4-217 shows facial and intraoral views on the second day after surgery. Usually, the most significant facial swelling occurs not on the following day, but on the second day. This patient presented with minor swelling of the face with no swelling of eyelids. Pressing the buccogingival transition zone led to the drainage of reddish exudate through the drain (yellow arrows on Fig 4-217b).

On postoperative day 4, the suture fixing the drain to the mocosa was removed and the drain was pulled out. Because the drain is made of silicon, removal is easy with no pain to the patient (Fig 4-218). The sutures were removed on postoperative day 7. Healing after surgery was favorable and the incision wound where the drain had been inserted closed spontaneously (Fig 4-219).

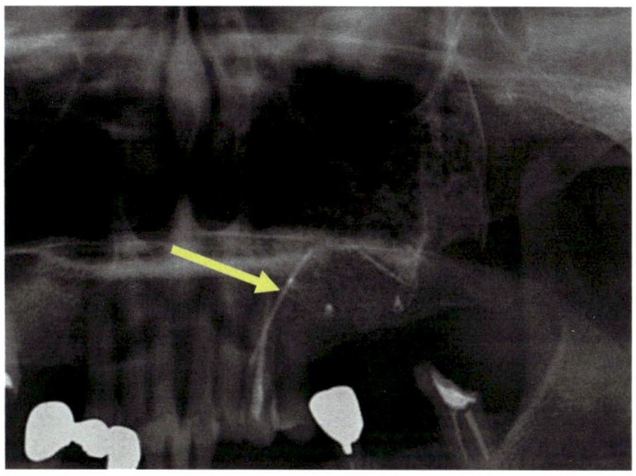

Fig 4-216 Panoramic view immediately after surgery.

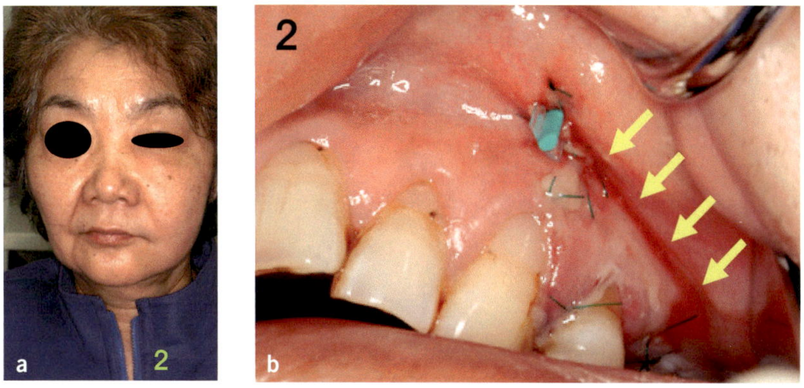


Fig 4-217 (a and b) Images on the second day after surgery.

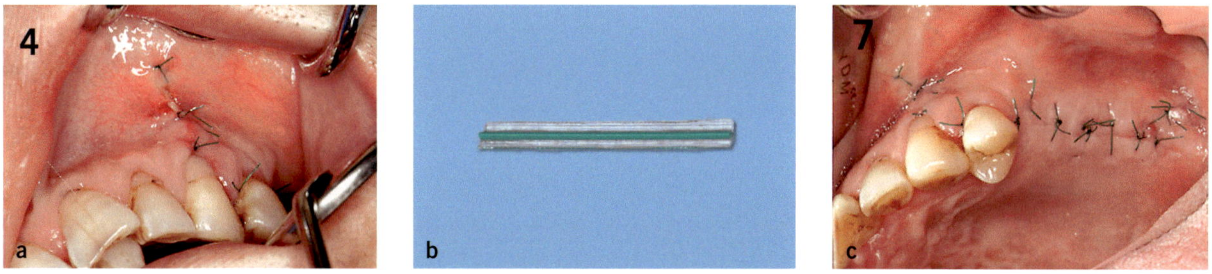


Fig 4-218 (a to c) Intraoral views on days 4 and 7, and the silicon drain.

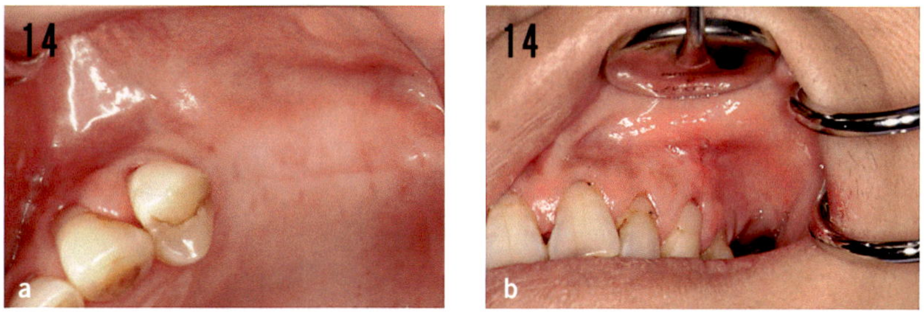


Fig 4-219 (a and b) Intraoral views on day 14.

## ! Key Point

This patient presented with minor swelling of the face but no swelling of eyelids. Pressing the bucco-gingival transition zone led to drainage of reddish exudate through the drain line.

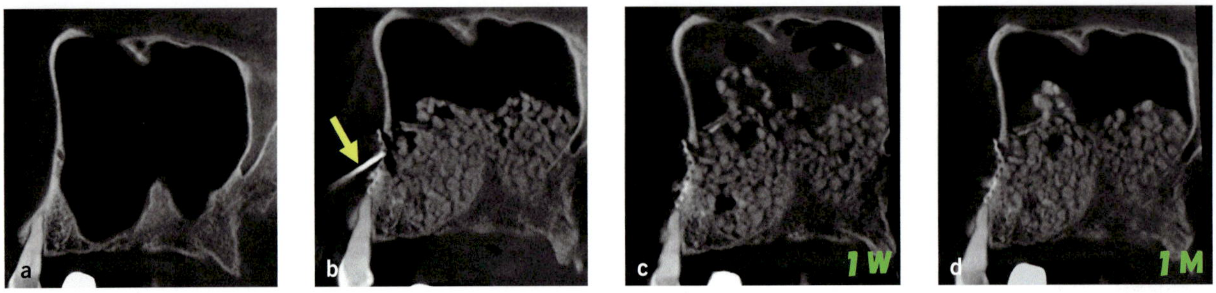


**Fig 4-220** CT images: (a) before surgery; (b) immediately after surgery; (c) at 1 week; (d) at 1 month.

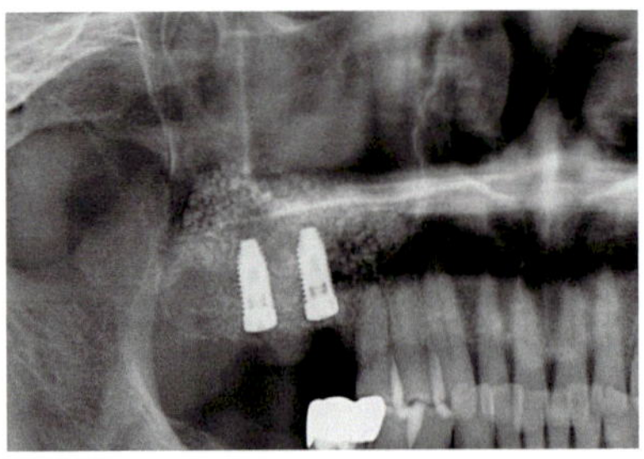

**Fig 4-221** Panoramic radiograph on first presentation.

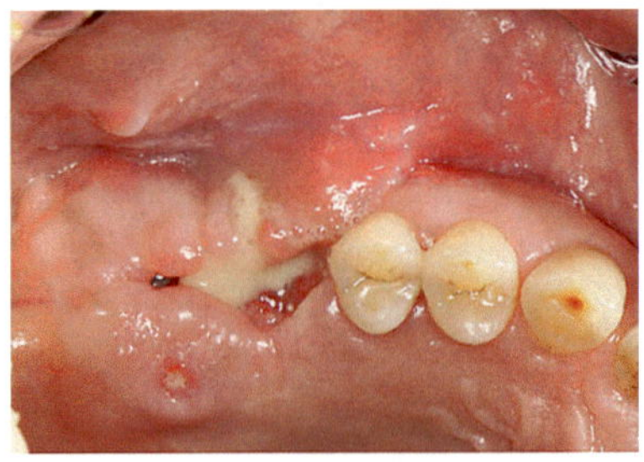

**Fig 4-222** Wound dehiscence at the crestal area of regions 16 and 17 on first presentation.

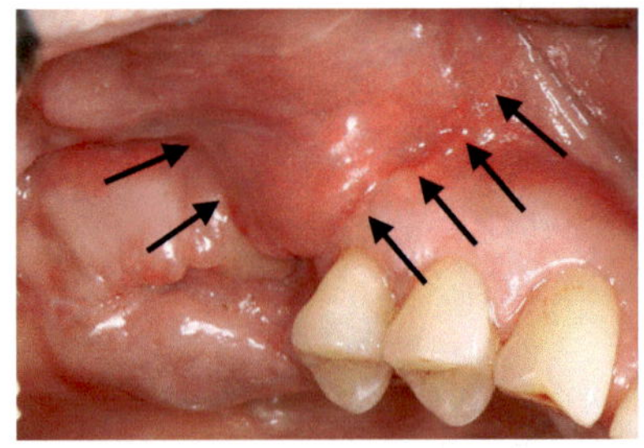

**Fig 4-223** Gingival swelling on presentation.

Figure 4-220 shows the postoperative CT images. Immediately after surgery, β-TCP granules were present in the augmented area and a radiopaque line of the drain can be seen (yellow arrow on Fig 4-220b). One week after surgery, a marked swelling of the maxillary sinus membrane was observed. One month after surgery, swelling of the membrane had disappeared and there was no noticeable loss of granules.

## Postoperative infection thought to be caused by swelling of the maxillary sinus membrane

Adverse effects of maxillary sinus membrane swelling, which occurs 1 week after sinus floor elevation, are not limited to the decrease of bone gain due to the dislocation of bone substitutes through the lateral window. There is also the serious risk that the dislocation of bone substitutes will lead to a dehiscence of the surgical wound and result in infection.

Should infection occur to the augmented sinus area, maxillary sinusitis would develop and necessitate removal of the bone substitutes. In such cases, deciding how much of the bone substitutes should be removed is difficult. The author first removes the material that has shifted from the augmented sinus area as well as loose material within the augmented mass. If the bone substitute employed consists of β-TCP alone, unnecessary granules are spontaneously eliminated by the body itself. On the other hand, in the author's opinion, if autogenous bone particulates have been mixed with β-TCP, the autogenous bone particulates will undergo sequestration and remain in the augmented sinus area as a heterologous protein, leading to prolonged inflammation.

### Clinical report 7: Pain and purulent discharge following sinus floor elevation

This patient was referred after undergoing extraction of teeth 16 and 17 2 months earlier, followed by implant placement with simultaneous sinus floor elevation about 3 weeks prior to the visit (Fig 4-221). According to the patient's treatment record, a mixture of autogenous bone particulates and β-TCP granules was used as the grafting material, no barrier such as a titanium mesh was used over the lateral window, the surgical wound was closed after making a release incision due to the immature mucosa around the extraction sockets of 16 and 17, and exposure of cover-screws, alveolar pyorrhea and pain occurred a week after surgery. Drug therapy and local irrigation could not improve the symptoms and the patient was sent to us.

Intraoral findings at the first visit included wound dehiscence at the crestal area of regions 16 and 17, with discharge of yellowish white pus from the buccal aspect of the dehiscence area (Fig 4-222). In the region from 15 to 16, gingival swelling was detected (black arrows on Fig 4-223), something

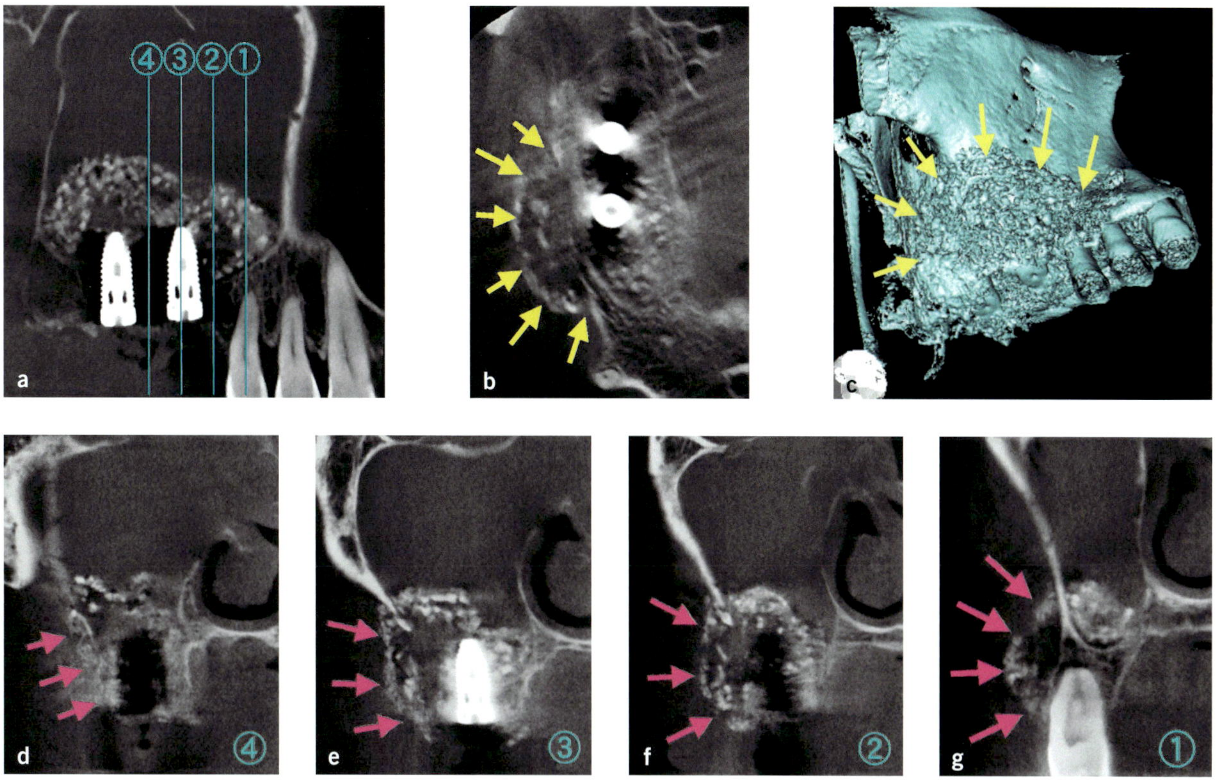


**Fig 4-224** CT scans at the first visit: (a) sagittal view; (b and c) horizontal and volume rendering images; (d to g) buccolingual views.

firm was felt immediately beneath the mucosa, and applying pressure to this area led to purulent discharge. Two implants at the regions of 16 and 17 and radiopaque granules in the augmented sinus area were observed on the panoramic radiograph.

On the sagittal CT scan taken during the first visit, radiopaque granules in the augmented sinus area and a marked swelling of the maxillary sinus membrane were observed (Fig 4-224a). Horizontal and volume rendering CT images revealed the buccal dislocation of the grafting materials through the lateral window (yellow arrows on Figs 4-224b and c). The buccolingual CT scan also indicated buccal dislocation of grafting materials in the area from the region of tooth 15 to the distal aspect of R1 (pink arrows on Figs 4-224d–g).

**! Key Point**

Remove the dislocated bone substitutes.

This patient was diagnosed with postoperative infection caused by the buccal dislocation of the bone substitutes. Treatment included removal of dislocated granules. These β-TCP granules were surrounded by granulation tissue and were removed carefully to prevent damage to the flap. Discolored autogenous bone particulates were found in the augmented sinus area and removed together with the loose granules (Fig 4-225). The granules that had incorporated into comparatively rigid soft tissue were left untouched. After irrigation, a drain was installed and the wound was closed.

After 3 weeks, swelling of the maxillary sinus membrane still remained but purulent discharge had stopped. Figure 4-226 shows the CT images obtained at that time. Despite continued swelling, dislocated β-TCP granules are no longer seen. Some granules incorporated into the soft tissue are visible around the implants, and these granules will be eliminated spontaneously once the body recognizes them as foreign substances.

Figure 4-227 shows intraoral views at 3 weeks after the surgery. No purulent discharge from the buccal gingiva at the region 16–17 was seen and gingival swelling at the region 15–16 had improved. Moreover, the patient experienced reduced pain of the right cheek. Careful follow-up will be necessary owing to the possibility of spontaneous elimination of β-TCP granules.

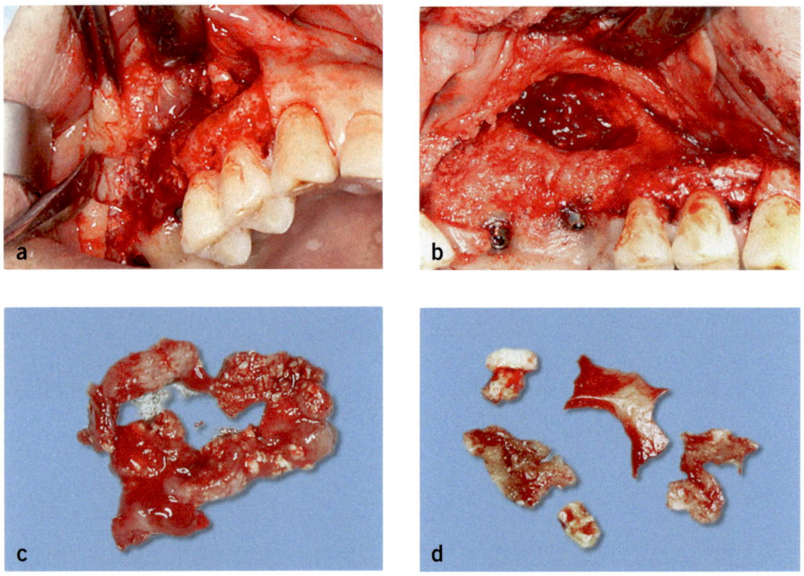

**Fig 4-225** (a to d) Removal of dislocated granules and autogenous bone.

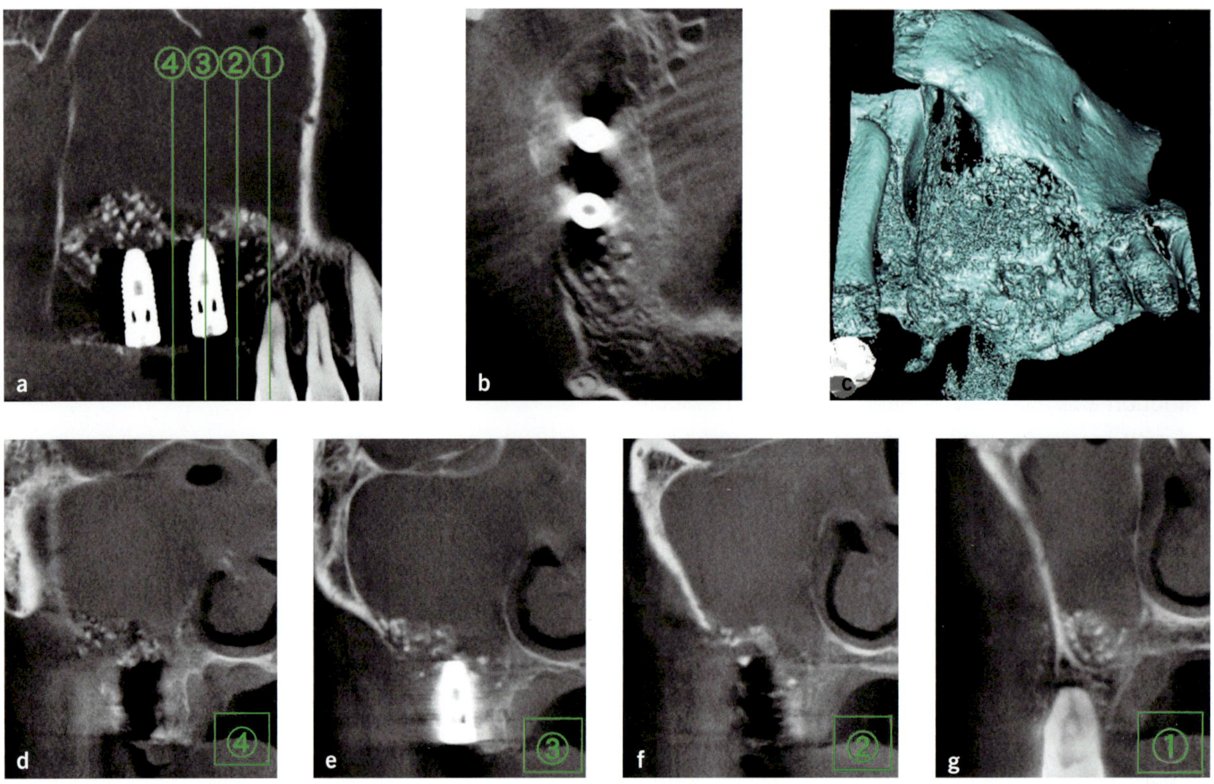

**Fig 4-226** CT scans 3 weeks after the surgery: (a) sagittal view; (b and c) horizontal and volume rendering images; (d to g) buccolingual views.

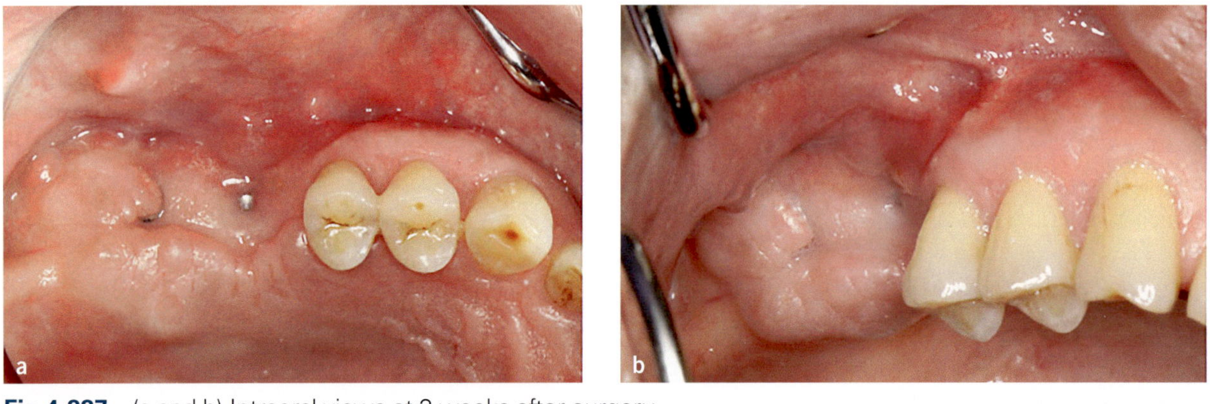

**Fig 4-227** (a and b) Intraoral views at 3 weeks after surgery.

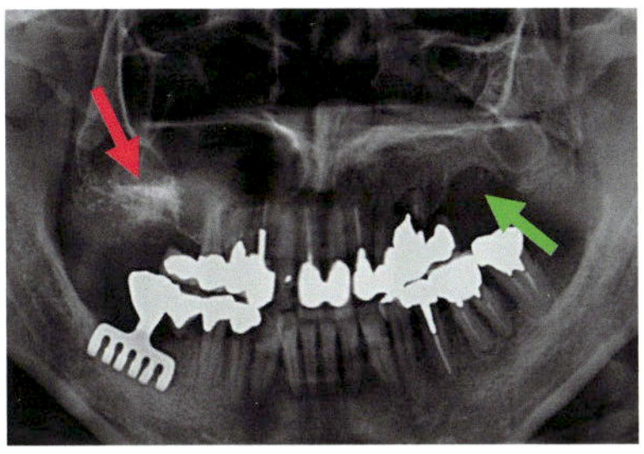

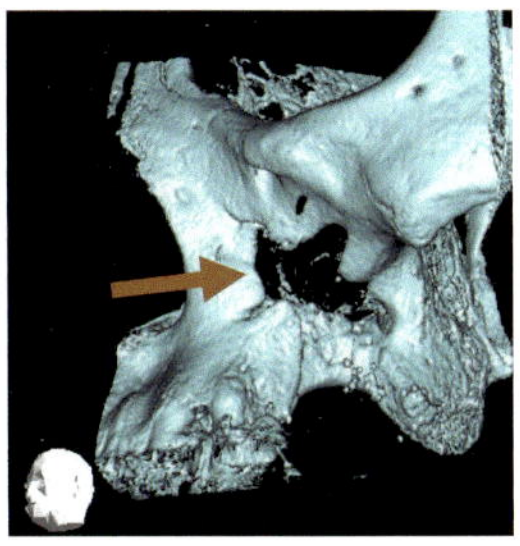

**Fig 4-228** (left) Panoramic view at first presentation.

**Fig 4-229** (right) Volume rendering CT scan at presentation.

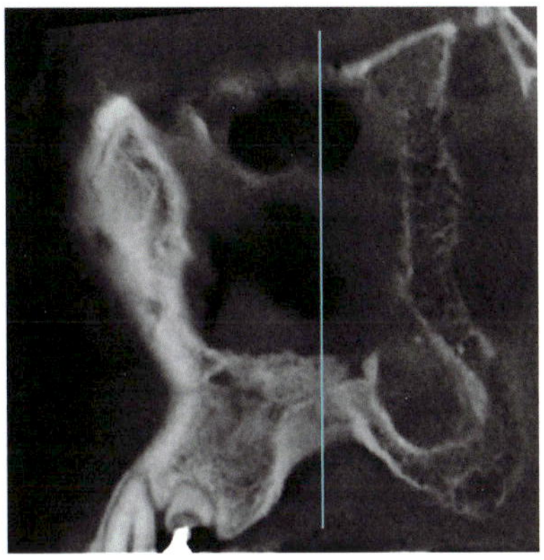

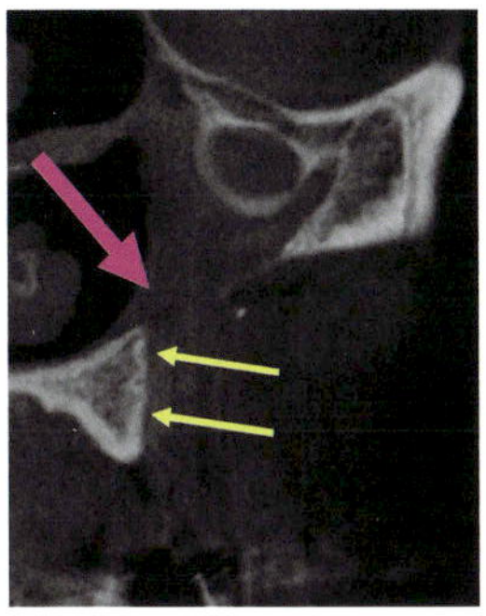

**Fig 4-230** (left) Sagittal CT image at presentation.

**Fig 4-231** (right) Buccolingual CT image at presentation.

## Laborious recovery from a failed sinus floor elevation

Infection after sinus floor elevation is often associated with maxillary sinusitis. If a patient with maxillary sinusitis consults an ENT doctor or an oral surgeon who does not provide implant treatment, it is possible that a radical surgical correction of the maxillary sinusitis will be provided. Because this type of surgery involves bone removal from the maxillary sinus anterior wall and the lateral wall of the inferior nasal meatus, the chance for another sinus floor elevation is lost. It will be challenging to explain this to the patient who possesses a strong desire for implant treatment. Therefore, prevention and solution of infection after sinus floor elevation is critical.

### Clinical report 8A: Marked bone defect making sinus floor elevation impossible

A radical surgical correction of maxillary sinusitis requires initial removal of bone from the maxillary sinus anterior wall followed by dissection of the maxillary sinus membrane. Next, the membrane and bone are removed from the lateral wall of the inferior nasal meatus to create artificial apertures.

The patient in this case was a 38-year-old female with a history of postoperative infection on the left side after bilateral sinus floor elevation. The patient had been treated with the radical surgical correction of the maxillary sinusitis on the left side at an ENT clinic. She now desired implant treatment in the upper left quadrant.

The panoramic radiograph at the initial visit indicated significant bone resorption at the alveolar crest in region 26/27 (green arrow on Fig 4-228) and a radiopacity at the right maxillary sinus (red arrow). A bone defect on the maxillary sinus anterior wall was shown by the volume rendering CT scan (brown arrow on Fig 4-229). From the buccolingual CT image it is evident that the bone had been removed from the lateral wall of the inferior nasal meatus (pink arrow on Fig 4-231).

The patient was fairly young and had a strong desire for implant treatment. However, taking into account the marked bone defect and scar formation in the area, bone augmentation was judged impossible.

**! Key Point**

It should be emphasized that treating postoperative infection after sinus floor elevation with radical surgical correction of the maxillary sinusitis will make another sinus floor elevation extremely difficult, if not impossible.

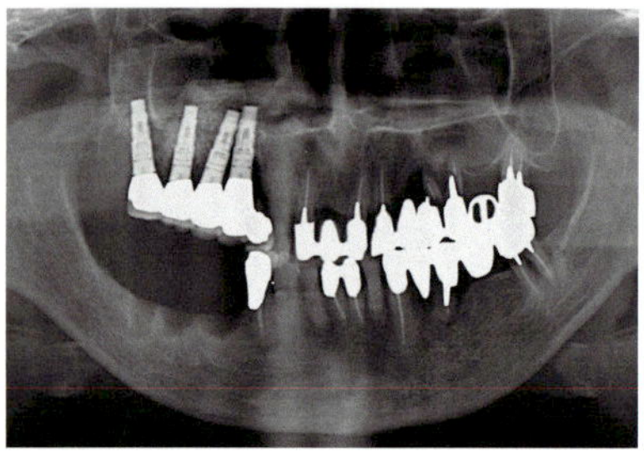

**Fig 4-232** Panoramic view at first presentation.

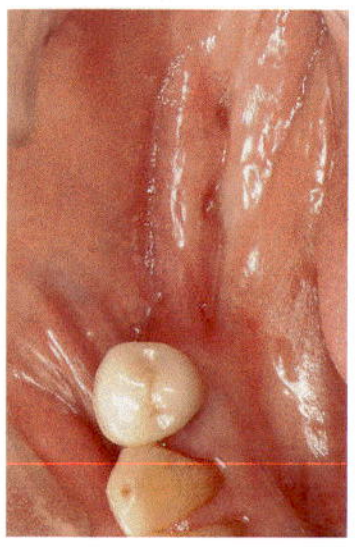

**Fig 4-233** Intraoral examination.

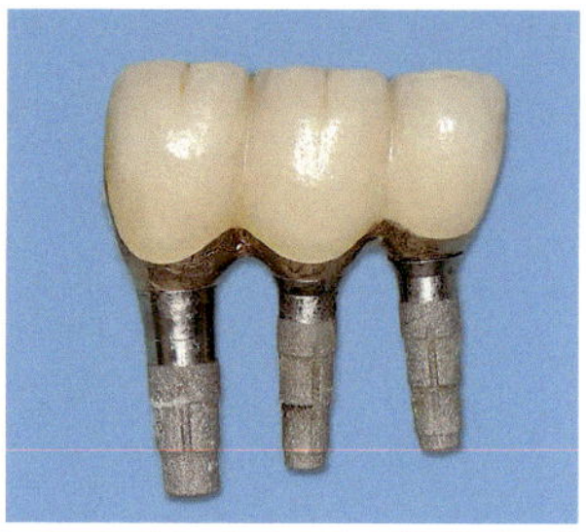

**Fig 4-234** The implants.

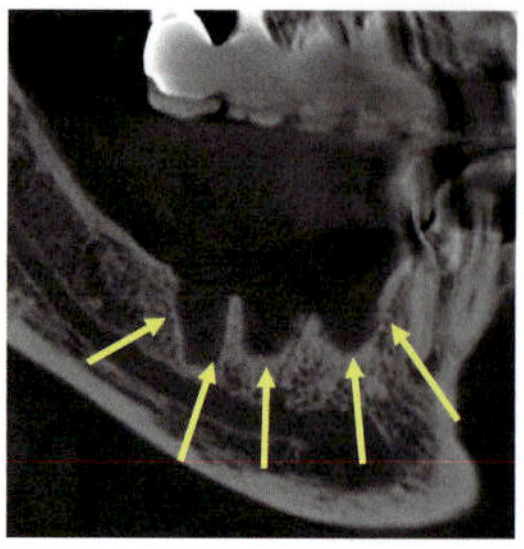

**Fig 4-235** CT image at first presentation.

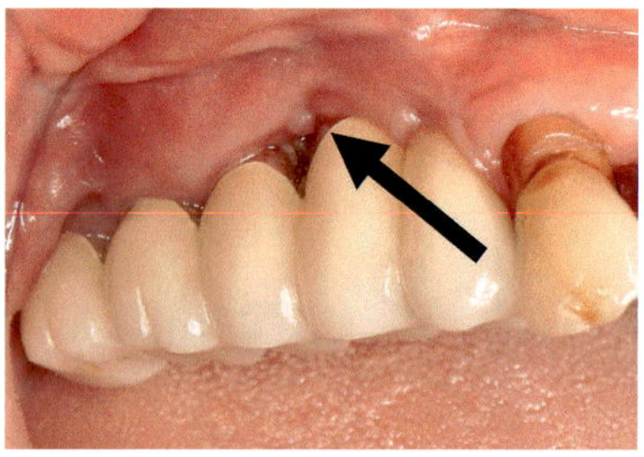

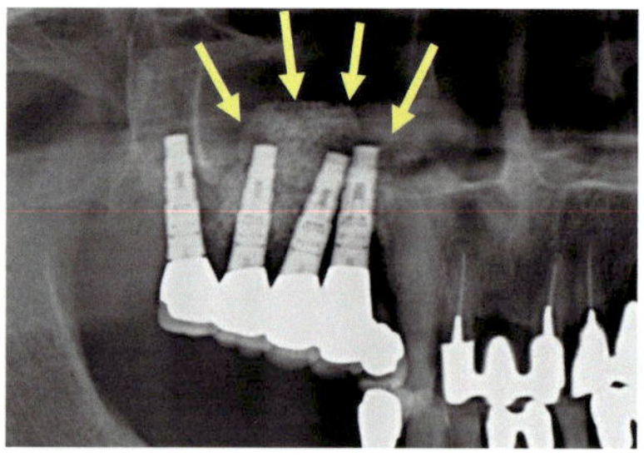

**Fig 4-236** (left) Intraoral view showing redness of the gingiva.

**Fig 4-237** (right) Panoramic view showing granule-like radiopacity around the implants.

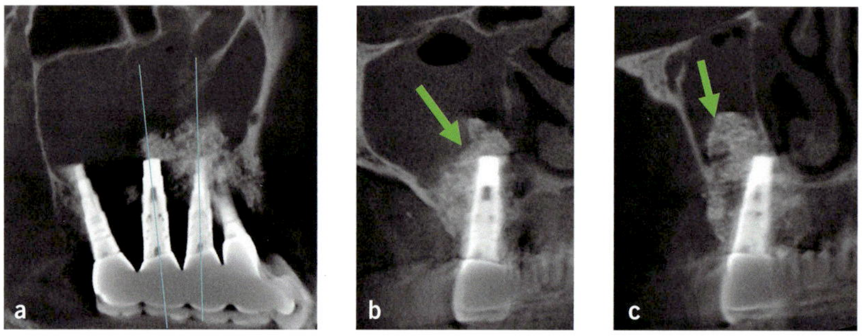

**Fig 4-238** (a to c) CT images of the implants in the maxilla.

## Clinical report 8B: Delayed infection after sinus floor elevation

This is a case requiring the removal of an implant and bone substitutes. The patient visited our clinic with the chief complaint of spontaneous loss of implants on the right side of the posterior mandible. The implants had been placed by the patient's regular dentist about 3 years earlier.

Intraoral examination at the first visit showed neither inflammation of peri-implant mucosa nor spontaneous symptoms such as pain (Figs 4-232 to 4-234). The radiopaque lines of the bone surfaces of the implant sockets were smooth (yellow arrows on Fig 4-235), which indicated that the implants had lost osseointegration long ago. This patient also had implants on the right side of the maxilla, which were placed 4 years earlier using sinus floor elevation and bone substitutes. Despite the absence of spontaneous symptoms, redness of the gingiva around R1 and R2 (black arrow on Fig 4-236) and mobility of implant superstructure were observed.

The panoramic radiograph showed four implants and granule-like radiopacity around the implants (yellow arrows on Fig 4-237). A marked swelling of the maxillary sinus membrane and granule-like radiopacity around the implants can also be seen on the CT images (green arrows on Figs 4-238b and c).

> **! Key Point**
>
> Clearly there is a risk of non-resorbable bone substitutes remaining in the tissue as foreign substances.

Although the superstructure presented mobility as a whole, there were no spontaneous symptoms. The patient was diagnosed with postoperative infection of the augmented sinus area and maxillary sinusitis on the right side. The implants and bone substitutes were removed under general anesthesia. No implant demonstrated osseointegration and every implant was easily pulled out by forceps.

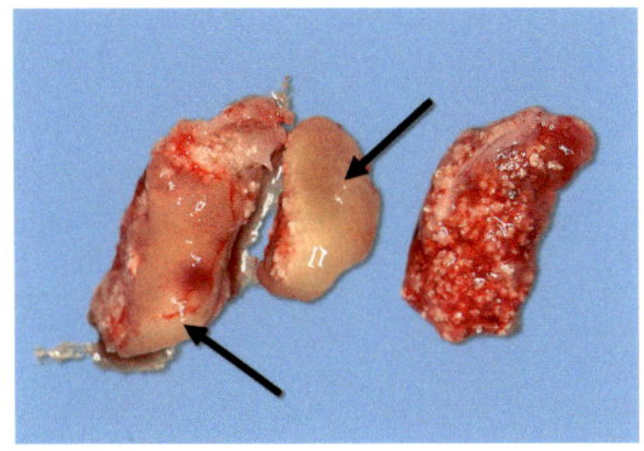

**Fig 4-239** The removed mass of bone substitutes.

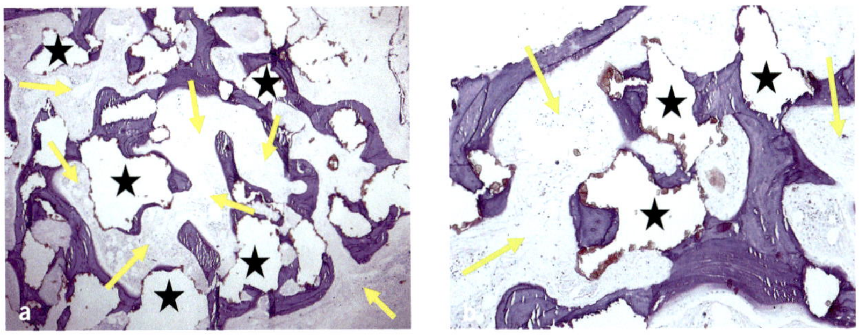

**Fig 4-240** (a and b) Toluidine blue staining of the removed bone substitutes.

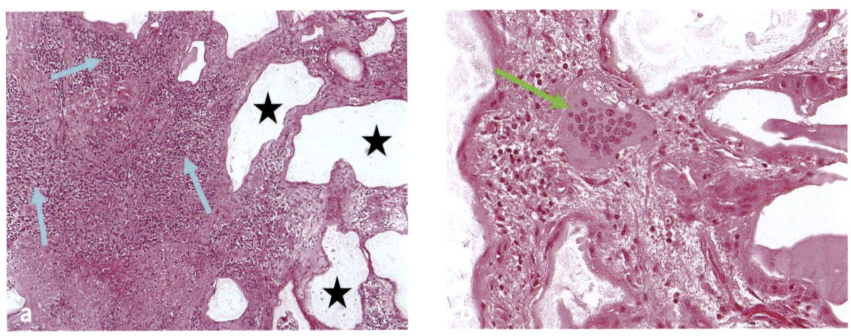

**Fig 4-241** (a and b) Sections of the removed mass (h&e staing).

Bone substitute granules had absolutely no mechanical strength, and even if they were forming a mass the hardness was similar to that of herring roe. After removing the implants and bone substitutes, the inside of the sinus cavity was irrigated, a release incision was made and the wound was sutured close.

The maxillary sinus membrane with edematous swelling adhered to the removed mass of bone substitutes (black arrows on Fig 4-239). On the histological evaluation sample stained by toluidine blue (Fig 4-240), bone stained in blue is observed around the bone substitute granules (marked with a star), but the soft tissue (yellow arrows on Fig 4-240) lightly stained by toluidine blue was present around the bone. Figure 4-241 shows the sections of the removed mass (h&e stained). Bone substitute granules (marked with a star) were surrounded by fibrous connective tissue in which infiltration of inflammatory cells (blue arrows on Fig 4-241a) and foreign-body giant cells (green arrow in Fig 4-241b) were observed.

**! Key Point**

There is a possibility that non-resorbable bone substitutes which remain in the tissue as a foreign substance may pose an infection risk over the long term.

Figures 4-242 and 4-243 show an intraoral view and CT image obtained 1 month after this surgery. Despite a sufficient release incision, an oroantral fistula remained (black arrow on Fig 4-242). Peri-implantitis existed at the time of implant removal and the inflammation of gingival tissue of the region was considered to be the cause of the remnant of oroantral fistula. Oroantral fistula (red arrow on Fig 4-243) and swelling of the maxillary sinus membrane were observed on the buccolingual CT scan, but the ostium was open (yellow arrow).

After the soft tissue around the fistula had stabilized, surgery was performed to close the oroantral fistula under general anesthesia (Figs 4-244 to 4-247).

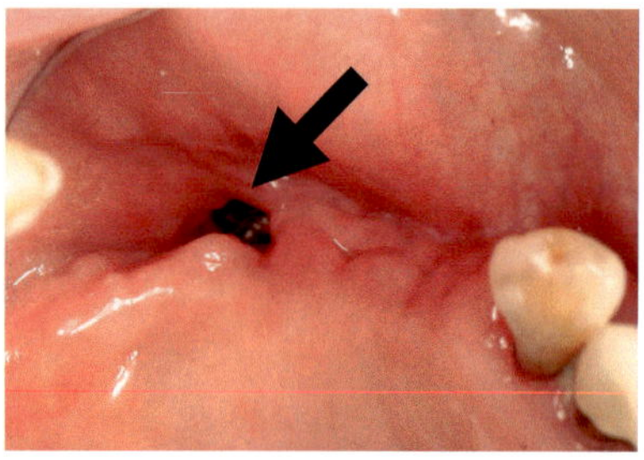

**Fig 4-242** Intraoral view 1 month after surgery.

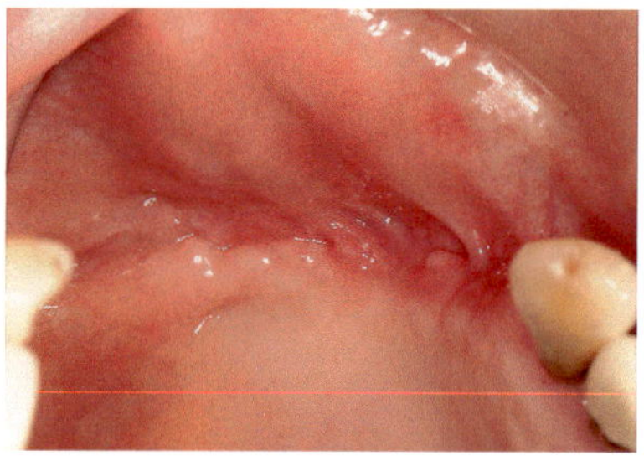

**Fig 4-244** Intraoral view 4 months after surgery, showing closure of the fistula.

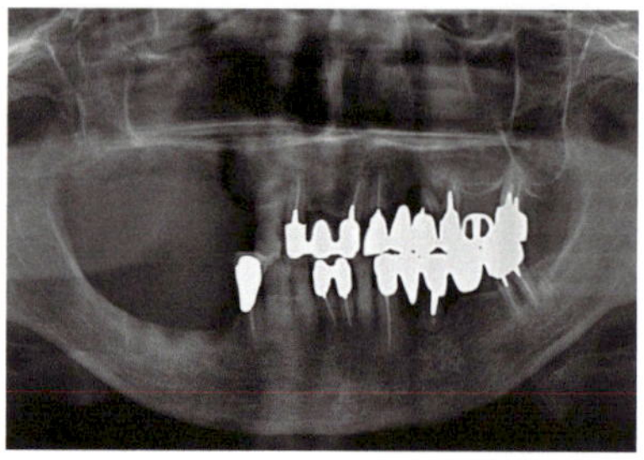

**Fig 4-246** Panoramic view 4 months after surgery.

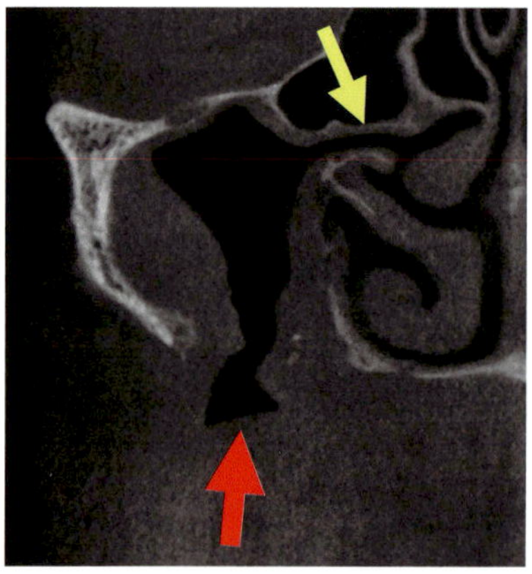

**Fig 4-243** Buccolingual CT image 1 month after surgery.

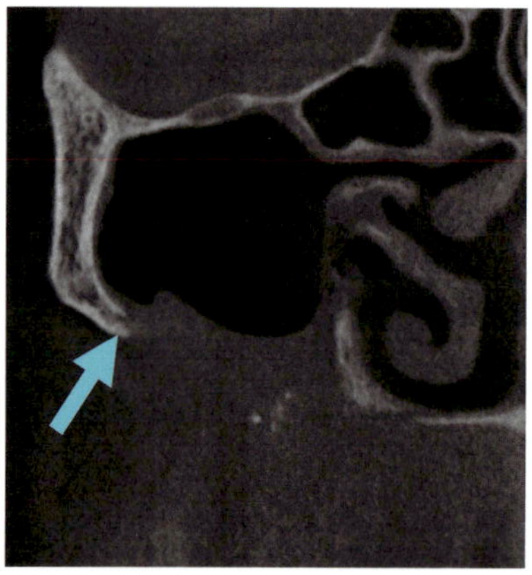

**Fig 4-245** CT image 4 months after surgery.

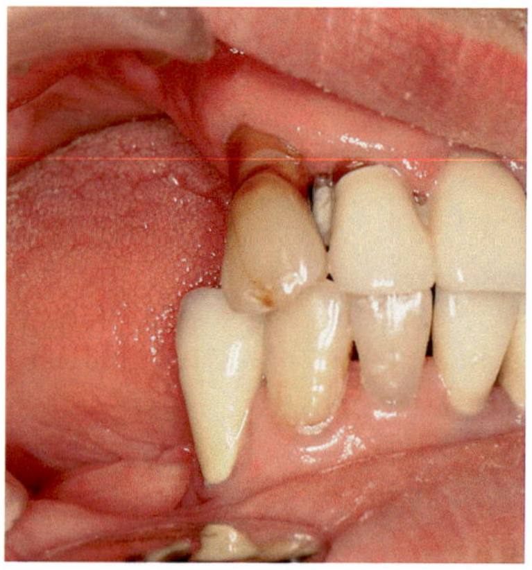

**Fig 4-247** The resulting extended alveolar defect.

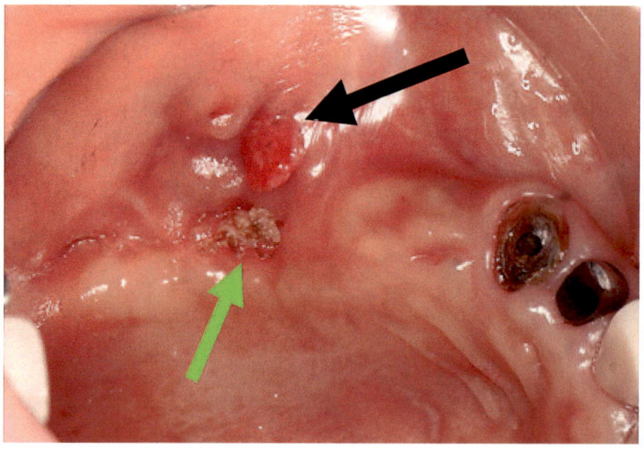

**Fig 4-248** Intraoral view at initial presentation.

The surgery included partial removal of the zygomatic process of the maxillary jawbone (blue arrow on Fig 4-245). Postoperative healing was uneventful; the oroantral fistula was closed and the swelling of the maxillary sinus membrane disappeared. However, an extended alveolar bone defect was left.

In this patient, the etiology of the infection of the bone substitutes was unknown. Because the superstructure was connected, the implant must have had osseointegration when the implants were restored. The occurrence of infection, however, caused destruction of the bone formed around the bone substitutes and resulted in the loss of osseointegration.

Though the cause still remains a matter of speculation, there is a possibility that non-resorbable bone substitutes which remain in the tissue as a foreign substance may pose an infection risk over the long term.

## Recovery from maxillary sinusitis after sinus floor elevation

When maxillary sinusitis develops after sinus floor elevation, elimination of the cause is the first priority. Patients often desire implant treatment even when they suffer from infection; therefore, the cause must be eliminated using the least invasive procedure while leaving open the possibility of another surgery for sinus floor elevation. In the patient to be reported next, the iliac bone marrow particulates, which contributed to the maxillary sinusitis and the edematous lesion on the maxillary sinus membrane, were removed, so that the option of a second surgery for sinus floor elevation was possible.

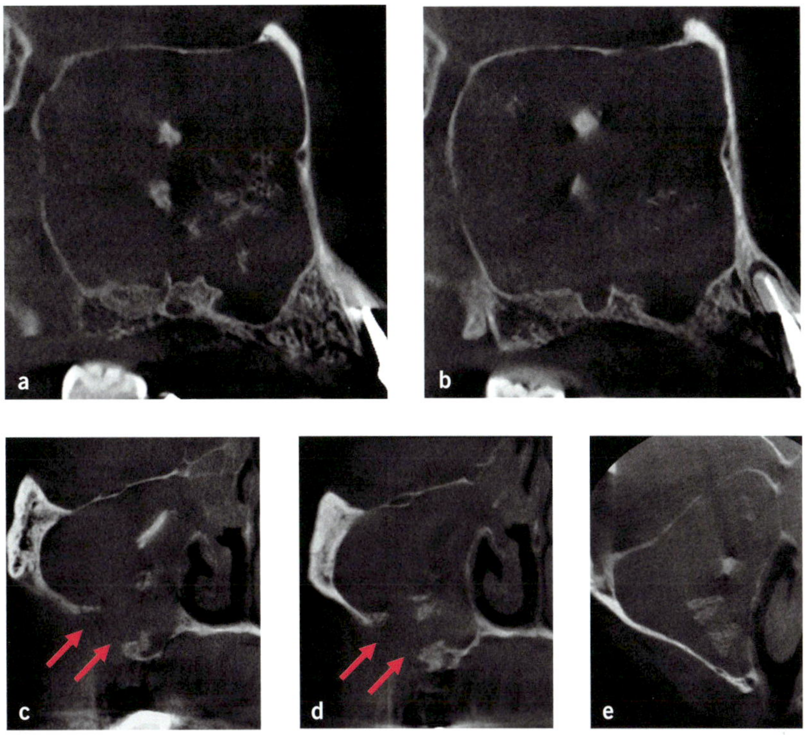

**Fig 4-249** (a to e) CT images at first presentation.

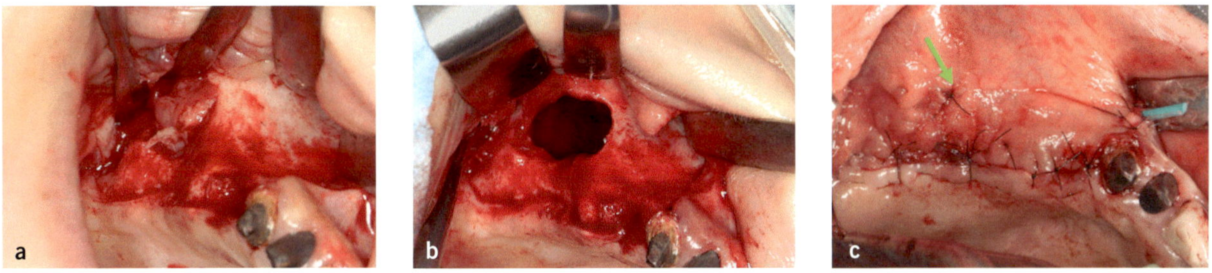

**Fig 4-250** (a to c) Intraoperative intraoral views.

## Clinical report 9: Example of recovery using a less invasive procedure

This patient had been treated at a hospital 3 months earlier with sinus floor elevation using iliac bone, and subsequently developed an infection. Because the hospital was far from the patient's home, she was referred to us.

At the initial examination, sequestrum (green arrow on Fig 4-248) and fistula (black arrow) were found, and the patient complained about dull pain in the cheek on the right side, nasal congestion, and heaviness of the head.

On CT images (Fig 4-249), the maxillary sinus membrane on the right side showed marked swelling, and radiopacity representing the bone particulates was observed within the maxillary sinus. The shape of the sinus floor was markedly uneven, and a bone defect, which is thought to have been the lateral window, was detected on the anterior wall of the maxillary sinus (red arrows on Figs 4-249c and d).

To begin the removal of the edematous lesion of the maxillary sinus membrane and sequestrum, a mucoperiosteal flap was created by sharp dissection at the area of the fistula and lateral window. Approaching through the lateral window, the edematous lesion of the maxillary sinus membrane and the sequestrum were removed. A drain was installed through the vertical incision and the fistula (green arrow on Fig 4-250c) and the wounds were closed with sutures.

Resected tissue was analyzed (Figs 4-251 and 4-252). In the soft tissue of the resected tissue, proliferation of dilated capillary vessels was observed immediately beneath the ciliated epithelium (black arrows on Fig 4-251c). Interstitial infiltration of inflammatory cells mainly consisting of lymphocytes and plasmocytes was observed (Fig 4-251d), which led to the diagnosis of chronic maxillary sinusitis.

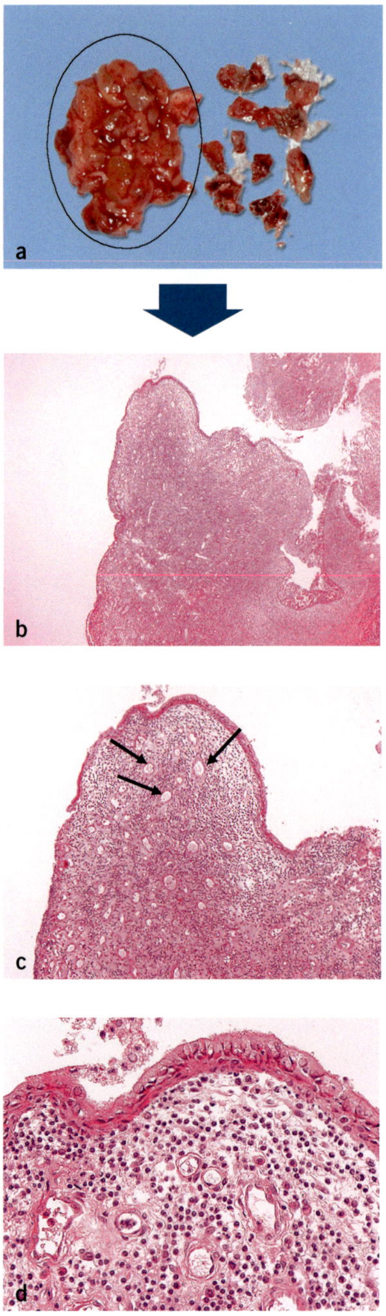

**Fig 4-251** (a to d) (left column) Histology of soft tissue.

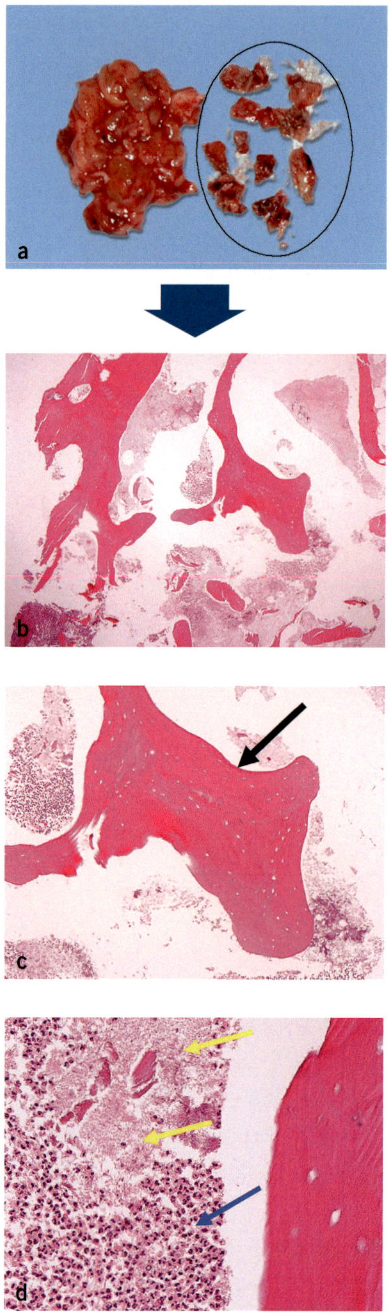

**Fig 4-252** (a to d) (right column) Histology of hard tissue.

The hard tissue removed was the bone tissue with unstained nuclei, later identified as the sequestrum (black arrow on Fig 4-252c). Infiltration of inflammatory cells, consisting mainly of neutrophils (blue arrow on Fig 4-252d), and the mass of bacteria (yellow arrows) were observed around the sequestrum.

> **! Key Point**
>
> The periosteum beneath the maxillary sinus membrane should be preserved to prevent postoperative bleeding. Only sequestrum and an edematous lesion of the sinus membrane were removed.

> **! Key Point**
>
> On the pathological section of the removed soft tissue, proliferation of dilated capillary vessels and infiltration of inflammatory cells were observed immediately beneath the ciliated epithelium. The resected hard tissue was determined to be the sequestrum.

Figure 4-253 shows an intraoral view and CT images obtained 1 year after this surgery. The fistula had disappeared and neither inflammation of the oral mucosa nor any symptom of maxillary sinusitis was found. On the CT images, swelling of the maxillary sinus mem-

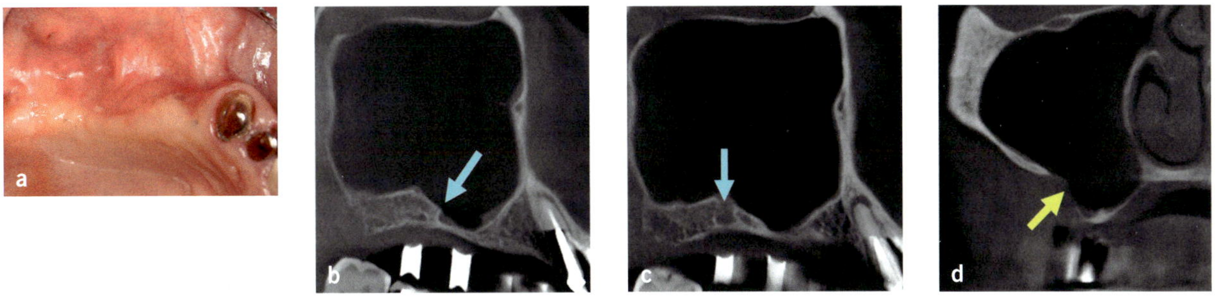


**Fig 4-253** (a to d) Intraoral view and CT images 1 year after surgery.

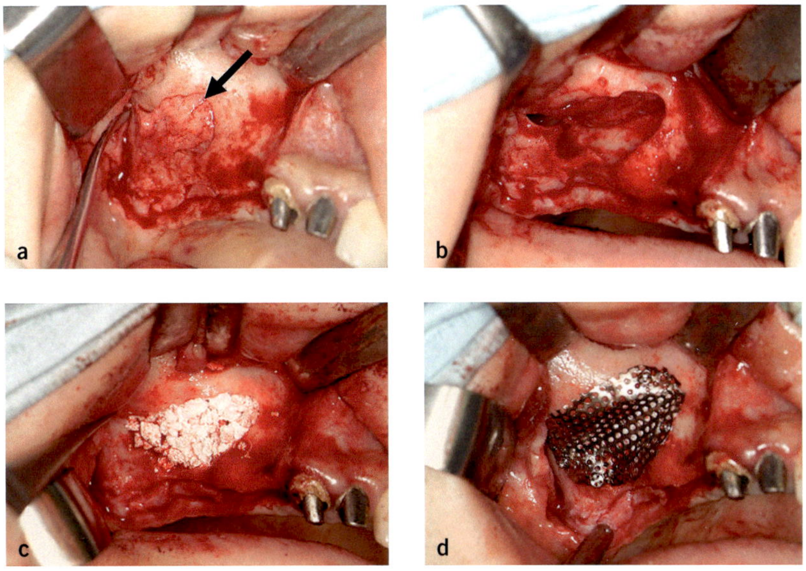


**Fig 4-254** (a to d) Second surgery for sinus floor elevation using β-TCP granules and titanium mesh.

brane was no longer observed, but the shape of the sinus floor was complicated (blue arrows on Figs 4-253b and c) with a bone defect on the maxillary sinus anterior wall (yellow arrow on Fig 4-253d). To meet the patient's strong desire for implant treatment, sinus floor elevation using β-TCP granules was performed.

There was a bone defect at the location where the lateral window was to be created. The mucoperiosteal flap was made using sharp incisions at the scar while avoiding damage to the maxillary sinus membrane (black arrow on Fig 4-254a). After elevating the maxillary sinus membrane and inserting the β-TCP granules, the lateral window was closed with a titanium mesh and micro-screws (Figs 4-254c to d).

> **! Key Point**
>
> Patients with a strong desire for implant placement often request a second surgery for sinus floor elevation, even if they have experienced failure due to infection of the augmented area. Therefore, recovery procedures that allow for a second attempt at sinus floor elevation should be chosen whenever possible.

The panoramic radiograph and CT images taken immediately after this second surgery for sinus floor elevation are shown in Figs 4-255 and 4-256. Though time-consuming, the maxillary sinus membrane was successfully dissected without perforation and the membrane on the medial wall could be sufficiently elevated. The β-TCP granules were situated immediately beneath the maxillary sinus membrane, and the radiopacity reflecting the titanium mesh was visible at the site of the lateral window (green arrows on Fig 4-256b).

The maxillary sinusitis of this patient was alleviated by extracting the sequestrum and edematous lesion of the maxillary sinus membrane, and a second surgery for sinus floor elevation could be performed. However, if this patient had visited a clinic where implant treatment was unavailable, the patient might have been treated with radical surgical correction of the maxillary sinusitis, a procedure where the membrane and bone of the lateral wall of the inferior nasal meatus are removed and an artificial aperture is created (yellow arrows on Fig 4-256b). The resulting creation of a bone defect on the lateral wall of the inferior nasal meatus makes sinus floor elevation, and thus implant placement, impossible. Therefore, should any problem occur relating to sinus floor el-

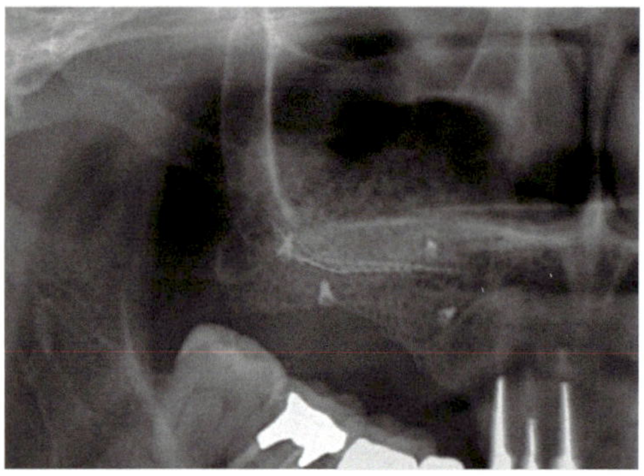

**Fig 4-255** Panoramic view immediately after second surgery.

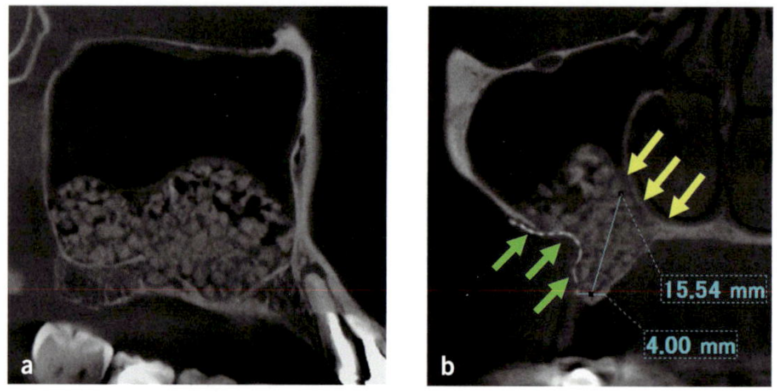


**Fig 4-256** (a and b) CT images immediately after second surgery.

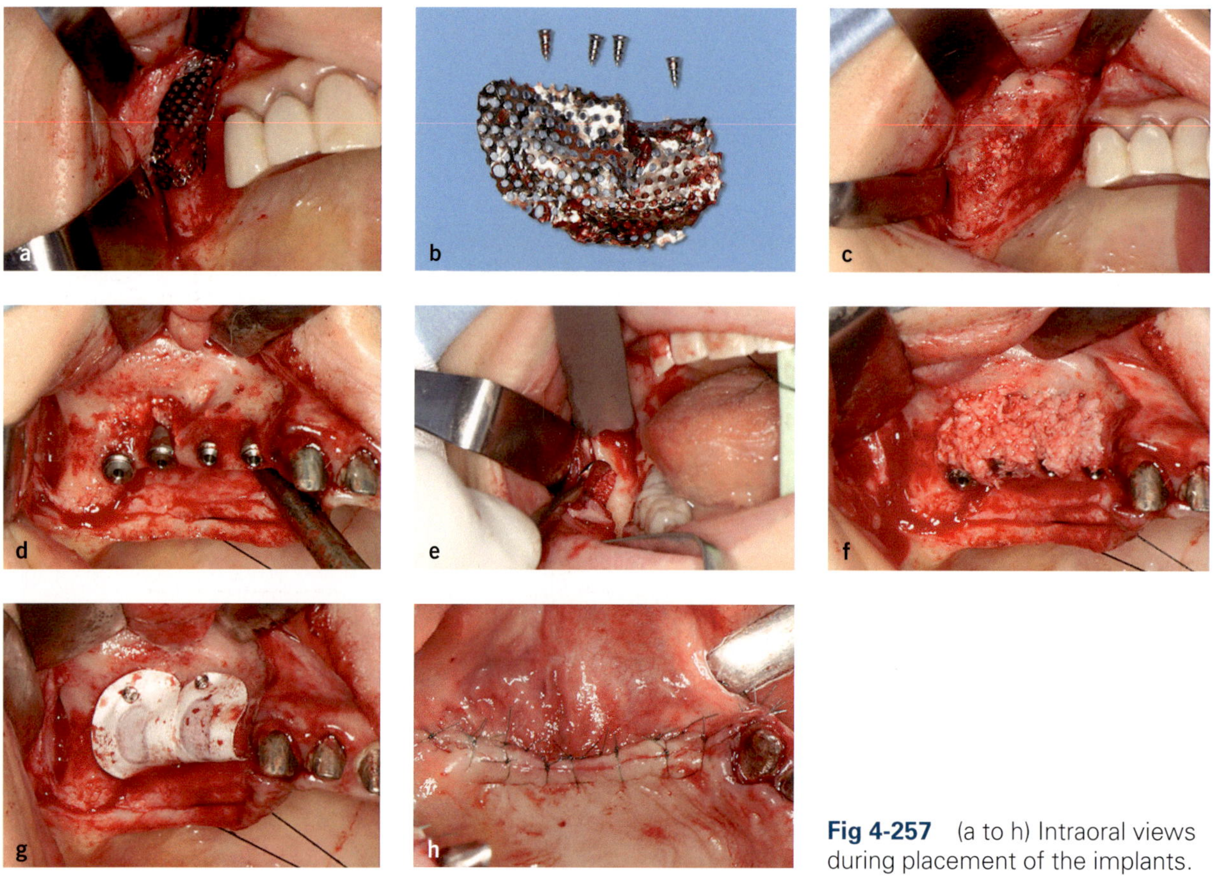

**Fig 4-257** (a to h) Intraoral views during placement of the implants.

evation, the patient should be referred to an oral surgeon with expertise in implant treatments.

In this patient, implants were placed 1 year after sinus floor elevation. When the titanium mesh at the lateral window was removed, some β-TCP granules had incorporated into the hard tissue (Figs 4-257a to c). Each implant achieved good primary stability. However, some exposure of the implants' surfaces was unavoidable owing to thin bone width (Fig 4-257d). Using the Easy Bone Shaver (Pro-Seed, Japan), autogenous bone grafts were harvested from the right ramus of the mandible (Fig 4-257e) and placed over the exposed surface. A non-resorbable membrane was placed over the implant site and secured with micro-screws (Pro-Seed, Japan) (Figs 4-257f and g). The wound was closed by making appropriate release incisions (Fig 4-257h).

**! Key Point**

Guided bone regeneration can be used during implant placement.

Figure 4-258 shows the panoramic radiograph and CT images obtained immediately after this surgery. The radiopaque line of the newly formed maxillary sinus floor can be seen (yellow arrows on Figs 4-258b to e), and there is no evidence of any swelling of the maxillary sinus membrane.

## Development of cortical and cancellous bones 2–3 years after surgery

The author uses either autogenous (iliac bone marrow particulates) or bone substitutes (β-TCP) alone. Both substances are eventually incorporated into the patient's bone and function as autogenous bone, provided the environment is favorable.

Postoperative follow-up after sinus floor elevation has revealed active modeling and remodeling up to 2 years after surgery. In other words, the augmented hard tissue is considered to be immature during the first 2 years, and consequently runs the risk, during this period, of easily changing to soft tissue depending on its microenvironment.

Hard tissue comprises cortical bone on the surface layer and cancellous bone inside. After 2–3 years of sinus floor elevation, the augmented area shows cortical- and cancellous-bone–like radiopaque lines, which indicates that the bone has stabilized. Therefore, the author believes that success and failure of sinus floor elevation can only be determined, by CT scanning, following this 2-year postoperative period.

### Clinical report 10A: Sinus floor elevation using iliac bone marrow particulates

This patient was referred for implant treatment within the maxilla. Based on the downward growth of the maxillary sinus observed on the preoperative helical CT, the patient was determined to require bilateral sinus floor elevation (Fig 4-259). The patient was informed about the differences between the options of grafting material, autogenous bone or bone substitutes. The patient chose to use autogenous bone, and the sinus floor elevation was performed using iliac bone marrow particulates.

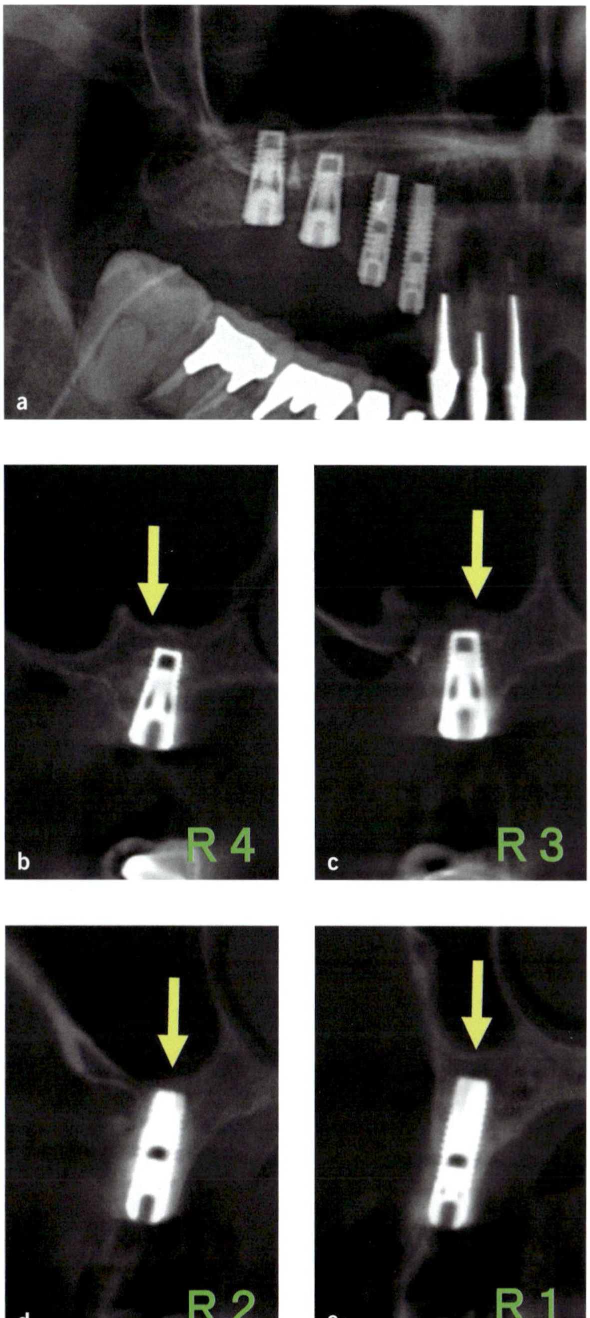

**Fig 4-258** (a to e) Panoramic view and CT images immediately after the surgery.

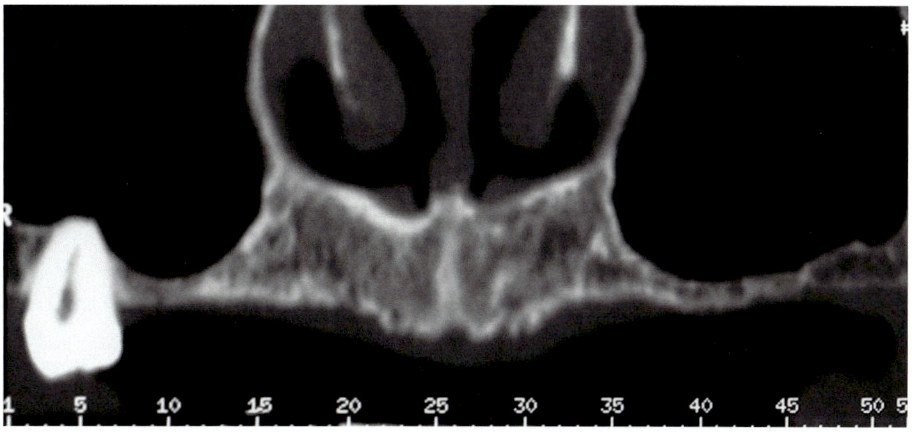

**Fig 4-259** Preoperative helical CT.

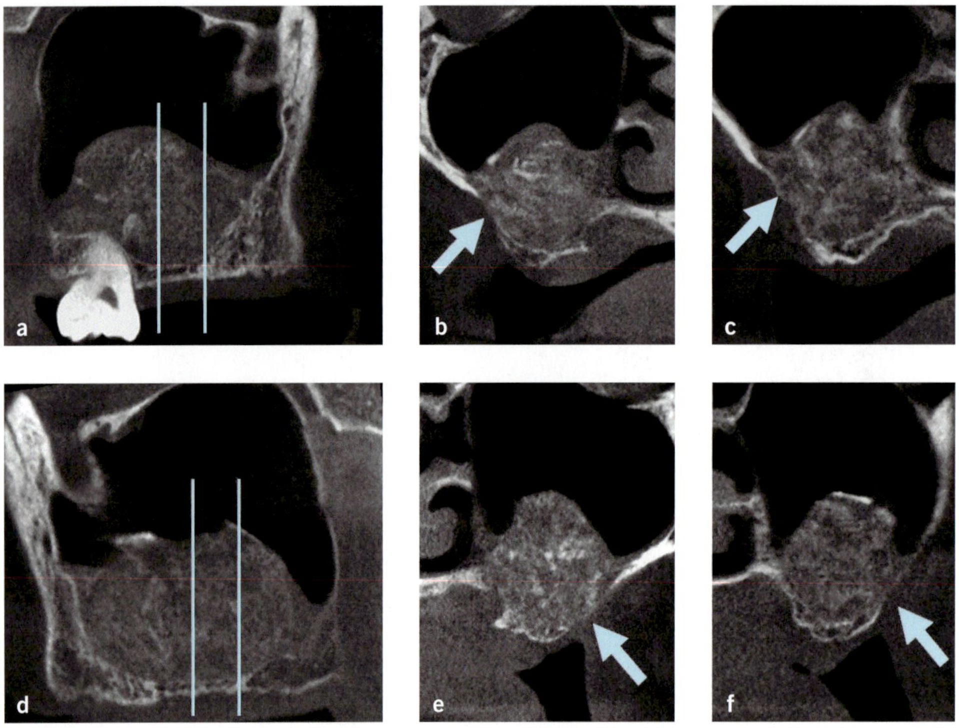

**Fig 4-260** CT images obtained 3 months after surgery: (a to c) right side; (d to f) left side.

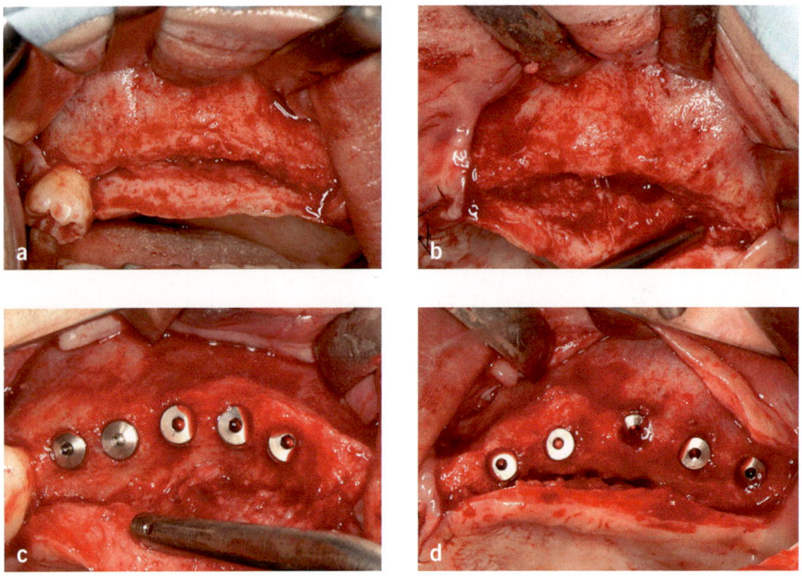

**Fig 4-261** Intraoral views during implant placement: (a and c) right side; (b and d) left side.

Figure 4-260 shows sagittal and buccolingual CT scans obtained 3 months after sinus floor elevation. The swelling of the maxillary sinus membrane is no longer seen, and irregularly shaped radiopacity, representing the autogenous bone particulates, can be seen in the augmented area. In the area of the lateral window, cortical-bone–like radiopacity was inadequately dense (blue arrows). Figure 4-261 shows intraoral views during implant placement performed 6 months after sinus floor elevation. Bone-like tissue was visually observed in the area of the lateral window and the border between the bone-like tissue and the native bone was unclear. Every implant achieved primary stability, but the bone quality during drilling was very soft. Figure 4-262 is a panoramic radiograph obtained immediately after implant placement. A total of 10 implants were placed and two Penrose drains were installed (blue arrows).

Figure 4-263 shows CT images obtained immediately after implant placement. The cortical-bone–like radiopaque line was observed along the lateral window (blue arrows); the radiopaque line of the newly formed sinus floor was observed only at R4 and R5 (yellow arrows).

Figure 4-264 shows CT images obtained 2 years after sinus floor elevation. A cortical-bone–like radiopaque line was observed along the lateral window and the newly formed sinus floor and had become

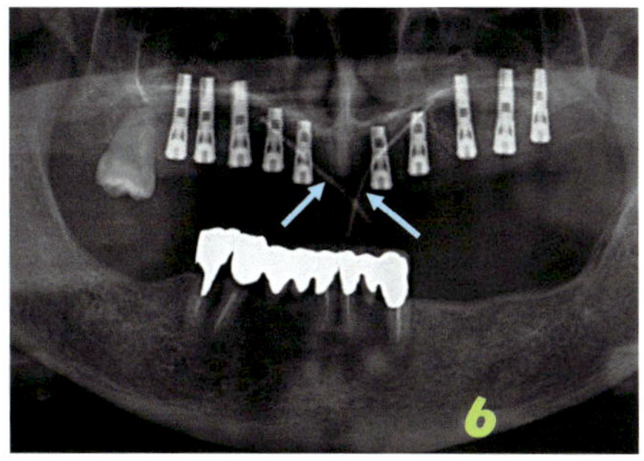


**Fig 4-262** Panoramic view immediately after implant placement.

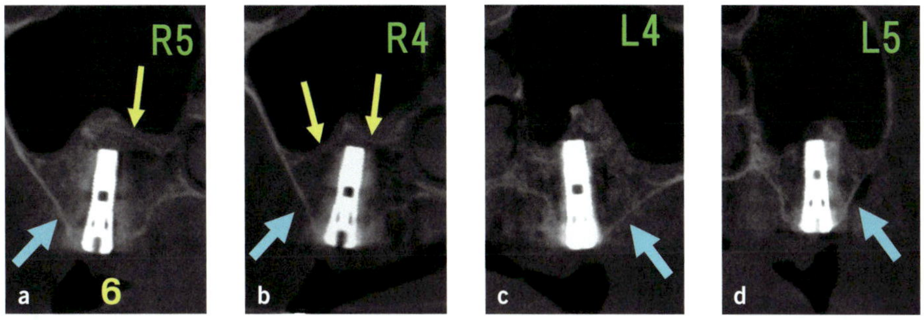


**Fig 4-263** (a to d) CT images immediately after implant placement.

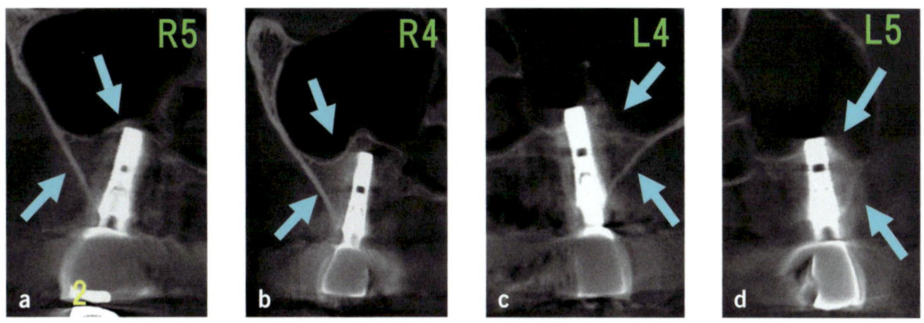


**Fig 4-264** (a to d) CT images 2 years after sinus floor elevation.

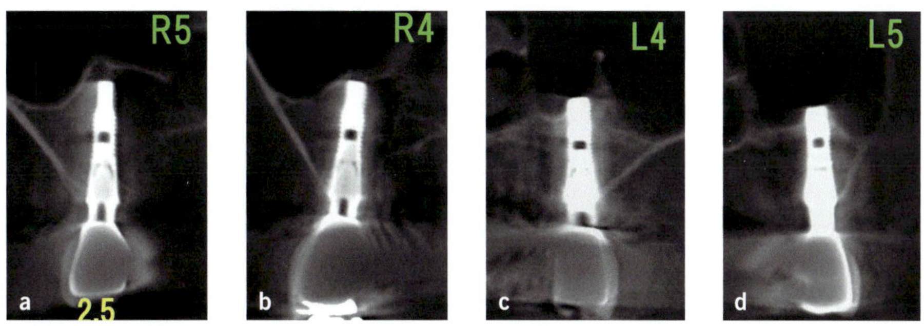


**Fig 4-265** (a to d) CT images 2.5 years after sinus floor elevation.

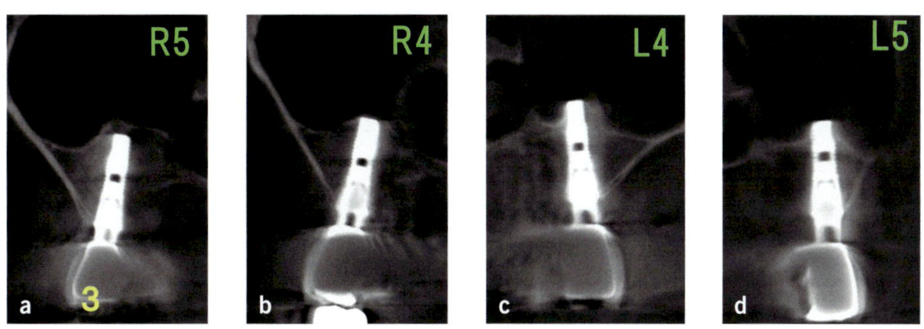


**Fig 4-266** (a to d) CT images 3 years after sinus floor elevation.

thicker (blue arrows). The interior of the augmented mass manifested a cancellous-bone–like radiopaque appearance. Thus the augmented mass was separated into cortical- and cancellous-bone–like radiopaque appearances.

Figures 4-265 and 4-266 show CT images obtained, respectively, 2.5 and 3 years after sinus floor elevation. The augmented site showed radiopacity similar to that observed 2 years after surgery, and was clinically stable.

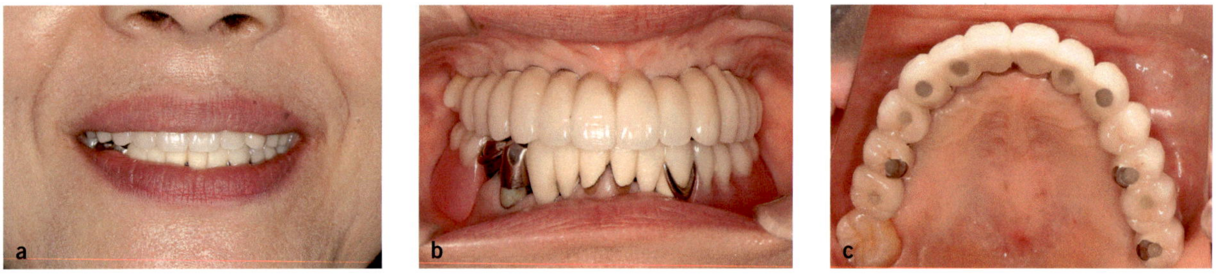


**Fig 4-267** (a to c) Clinical images 3 years after sinus floor elevation.

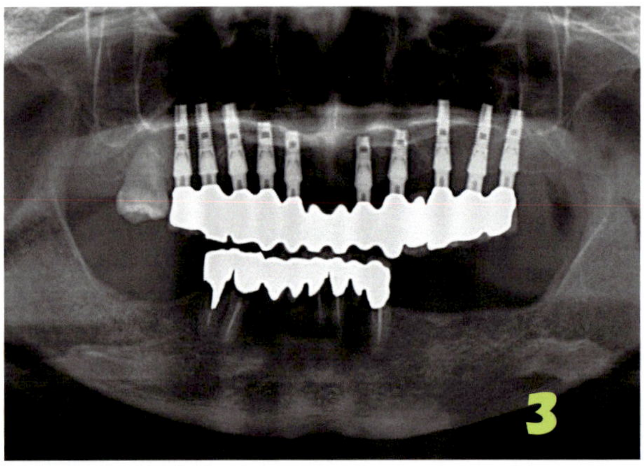


**Fig 4-268** Panoramic view 3 years after sinus floor elevation.

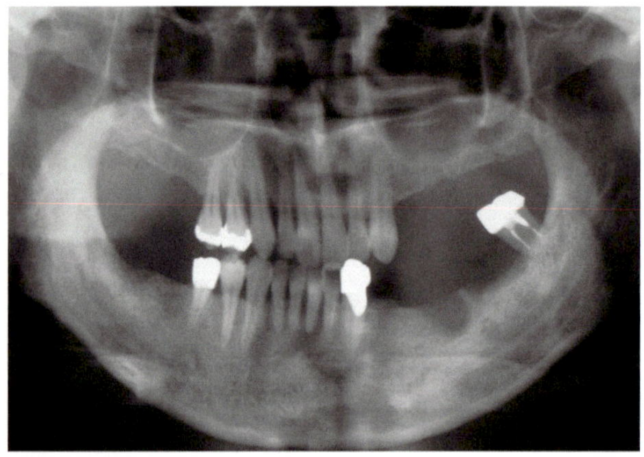

**Fig 4-269** Panoramic view on referral.

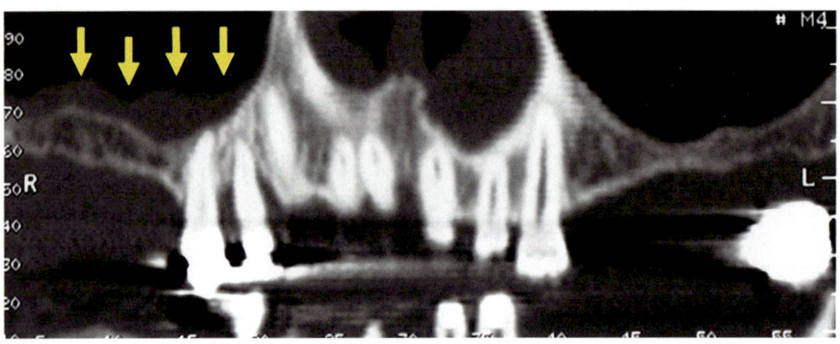


**Figs 4-270** Helical CT on referral.

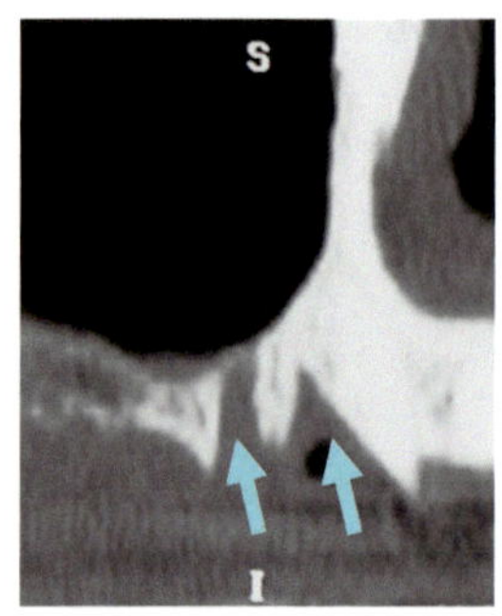


**Fig 4-271** CT image 3 months after extraction of teeth 14 and 15.

Figure 4-267 shows facial and intraoral views obtained 3 years after the sinus floor elevation. Screw-retained superstructures were connected to the implants, and the patient's satisfaction was very high (Fig 4-267). A panoramic radiograph demonstrated stable vertical bone levels (Fig 4-268).

## Clinical report 10B: Sinus floor elevation using iliac bone marrow particulates

This patient was referred for implant treatment in the bilateral posterior maxilla (Fig 4-269). Preoperative helical CT revealed swelling of the maxillary sinus membrane (yellow arrows on Fig 4-270) and mobility of teeth 14 and 15 with bone resorption in that area.

On the CT image obtained 3 months after the extraction of teeth 14 and 15, osseous healing of the extraction sockets was seen to be incomplete (blue arrows on Fig 4-271), but the swelling of the maxillary sinus membrane had disappeared. Therefore, sinus floor elevation using iliac bone marrow particulates was performed.

After the creation of a lateral window on each side of the maxillary sinus anterior wall, the maxillary sinus membrane was elevated and iliac bone marrow particulates were placed into the space (yellow arrows on Figs 4-272a and b). The extraction sockets (blue arrows on Figs 4-272a) of 14 and 15 were also filled with the bone particulates and the wound was closed. Implant

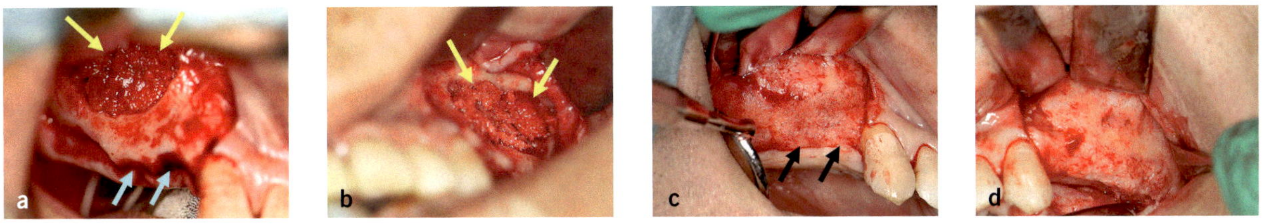

**Fig 4-272** (a and b) Intraoperative intraoral images. (c and d) Intraoperative intraoral images during implant placement.

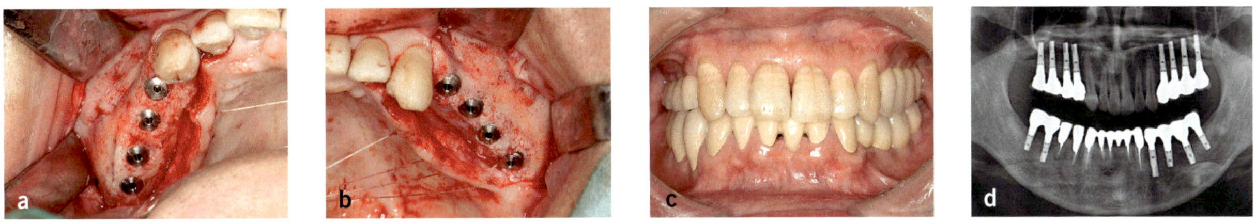

**Fig 4-273** (a and b) Implant placement: during sinus floor elevation. (c and d) Intraoral and radiographic image after fabrication of the superstructures.

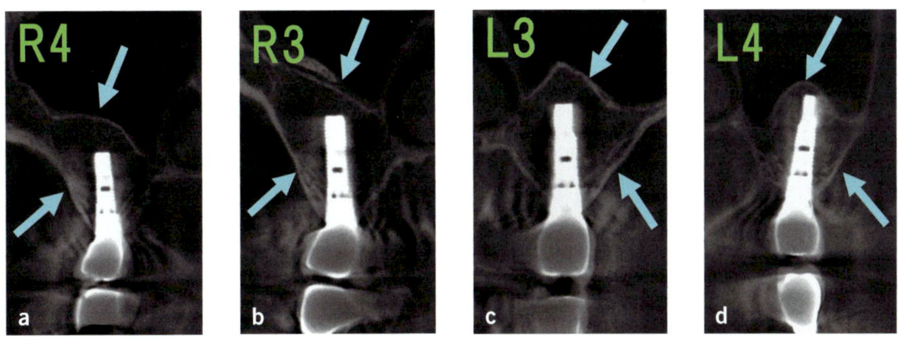


**Fig 4-274** (a to d) CT images 2.5 years after sinus floor elevation.

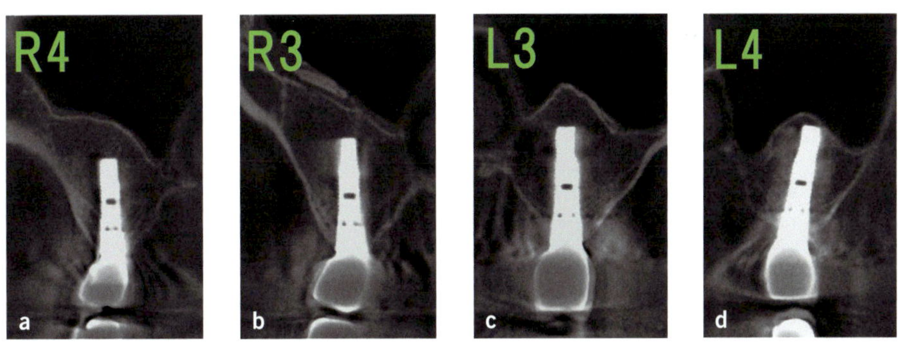


**Fig 4-275** (a to d) CT images 5 years after sinus floor elevation.

placement was performed 6 months after sinus floor elevation. Bone-like tissue was visually observed in the area of the lateral window, and the border between the bone-like tissue and the native bone was unclear (Figs 4-272c and d). The bone particulates used to fill the extraction sockets had transformed to resemble bone-like tissue (black arrows on Fig 4-272c).

Four implants were placed in the posterior region of each quadrant of the maxilla (Figs 4-273a and b). Every implant achieved osseointegration and the superstructures were prepared and connected by the patient's regular dentist (Figs 4-273c and d). Postoperative follow-up was performed in collaboration with the patient's regular dentist.

Radiopacity was observed at the augmented area on the buccolingual CT image 2.5 years after sinus floor elevation, being separated into cortical- and cancellous-bone–like radiopaque appearances (blue arrows on Fig 4-274). The buccolingual CT image 5 years after surgery was similar, was clinically stable (Fig 4-275).

## Clinical report 10C: Sinus floor elevation using iliac bone marrow particulates

This patient was referred for implant treatment on the left side of the posterior maxilla (Fig 4-276). Preoperative helical CT revealed the presence of three septa (yellow arrows on Fig 4-277) and slight swell-

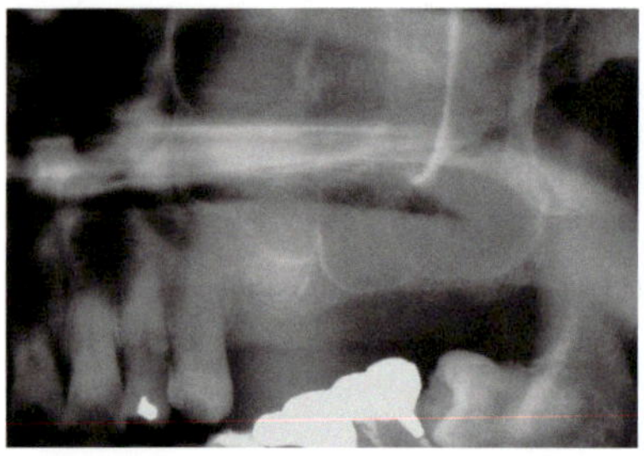

**Fig 4-276** (left) Panoramic view on referral.

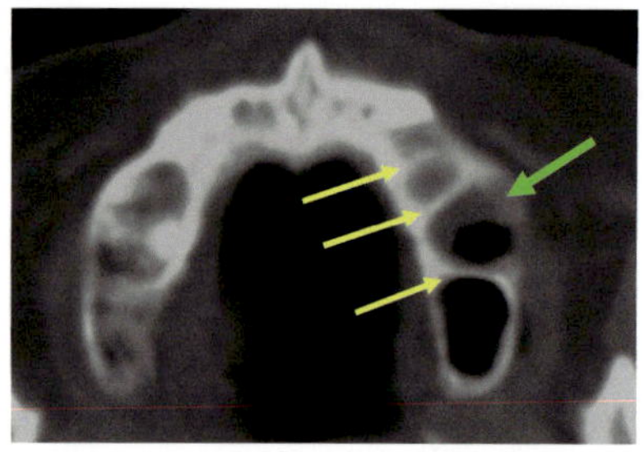

**Fig 4-277** (right) Helical CT before surgery.

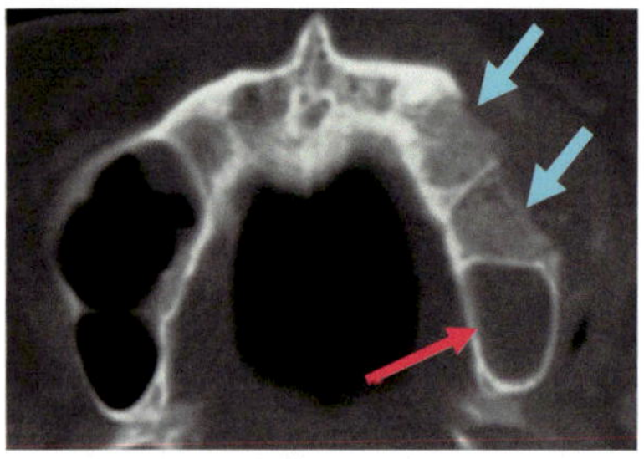

**Fig 4-278** (left) Helical CT 2 weeks after surgery.

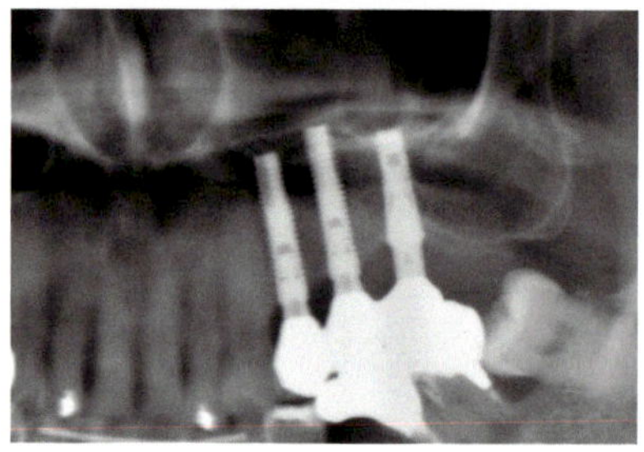

**Fig 4-279** (right) Panoramic image 6 years after surgery.

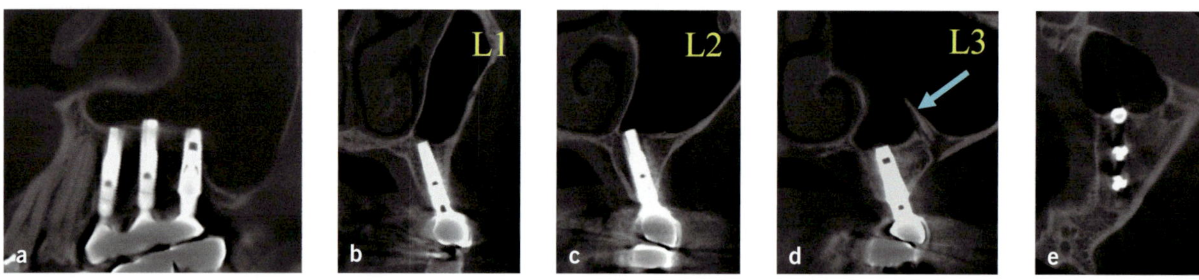


**Fig 4-280** (a to e) CT images 6 years after surgery.

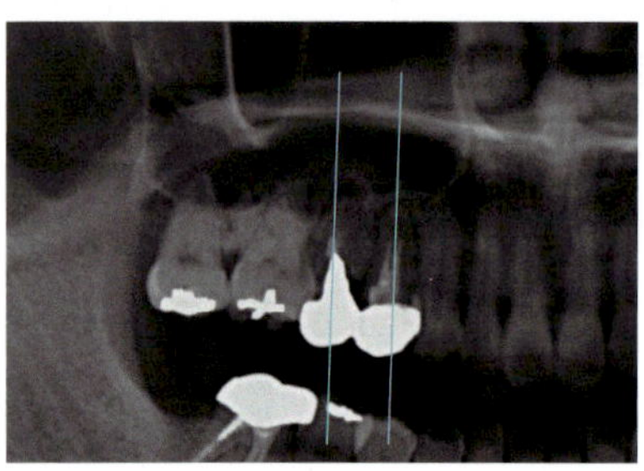

**Fig 4-281** Panoramic view on referral.

ing of the maxillary sinus membrane (green arrow). Sinus floor elevation using iliac bone marrow particulates was performed (blue arrows on Fig 4-278) except for the distal region of the most posterior septum. Swelling of the maxillary sinus membrane was observed posterior to the septum on the CT image 2 weeks after the operation (red arrow).

> **! Key Point**
>
> Swelling of the maxillary sinus membrane was observed posterior to the septum on the CT image 2 weeks postoperatively (red arrow on Fig 4-278).

Figures 4-279 and 4-280 show images obtained 6 years after the surgery. Sufficient radiopacity was observed around implants, and the radiopacity at the augmented area was separated into cortical- and cancellous-bone–like radiopaque appearances. The distal part of L3 was in close proximity to the maxillary sinus, but no sign of inflammation was found to the maxillary sinus membrane. A radiopacity, which was considered to represent the lateral window, can be seen in the upper buccal area of L3 (blue arrow on Fig 4-280d).

> **! Key Point**
>
> The region augmented by iliac bone marrow particulates showed cortical- and cancellous-bone–like radiopaque appearances on the CT images taken 6 years after surgery and was clinically stable.

## Clinical report 11A: Sinus floor elevation using β-TCP alone

This patient visited us with the chief complaint of mobility of teeth 14 and 15 (Fig 4-281). Root frac-

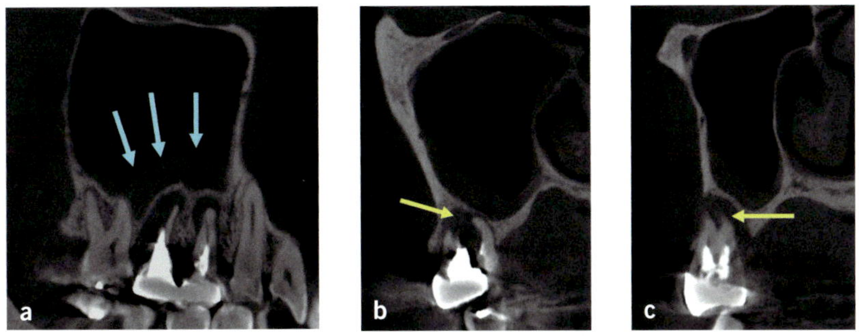


Fig 4-282 (a to c) CT images on referral.

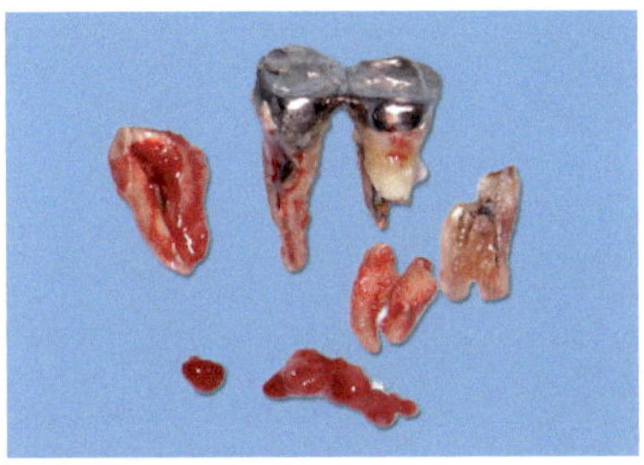

Fig 4-283 Extracted teeth and granulation tissues.

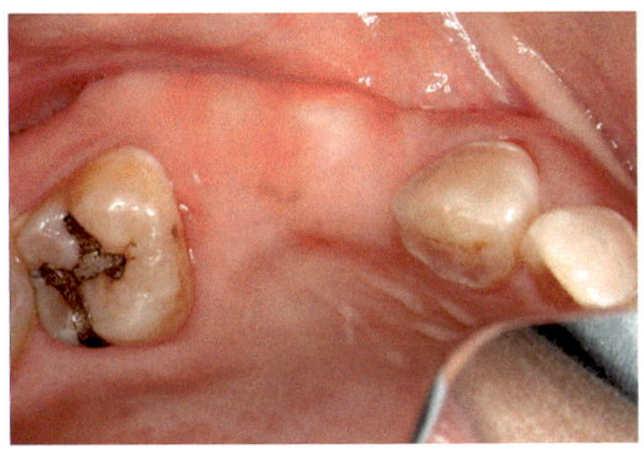

Fig 4-284 Intraoral view 5 months after surgery.

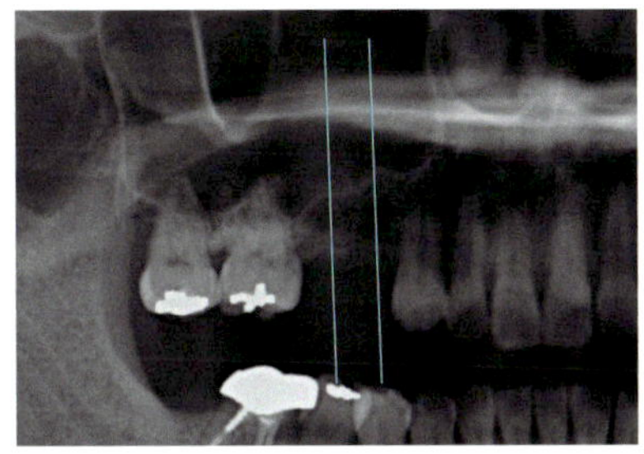

Fig 4-285 Panoramic view 5 months after surgery.

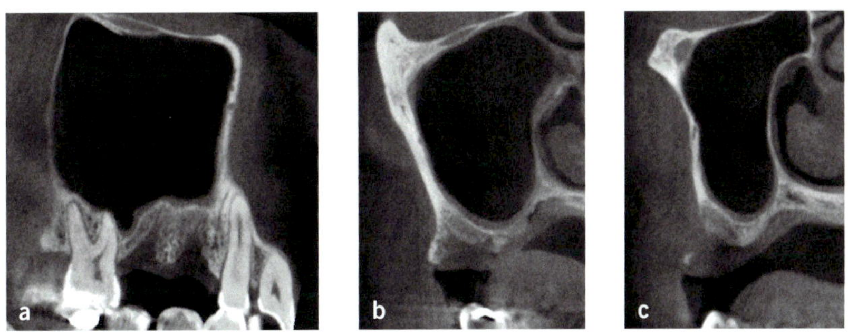


Fig 4-286 (a to c) CT images 5 months after surgery.

ture of teeth 14 and 15 and bone resorption within this region were observed on the CT image taken during the first visit (yellow arrows on Figs 4-282b and c). Swelling of the maxillary sinus membrane at the region of teeth 14 and 15 was also observed (blue arrows on Fig 4-282a). Teeth 14 and 15 as well as unfavorable granulation tissues were removed (Fig 4-283).

Figures 4-284 and 4-285 are intraoral and panoramic views 5 months after this surgery. On the CT images, the swelling of the sinus membrane had disappeared but bone regeneration in the extraction socket was inadequate (Fig 4-286). Because the oral mucosa had already healed, sinus floor elevation and simultaneous GBR using β-TCP were performed.

Figure 4-287 shows a series of intraoral views obtained during the bone augmentation surgery. After thorough debridement of extraction sockets, a lateral window was created using a diamond round bur. After elevating the maxillary sinus membrane, the space under the elevated sinus membrane and the extraction sockets were filled with β-TCP and closed by covering with a non-resorbable barrier membrane.

The barrier membrane was removed 1 year after the bone augmentation and implants were inserted (Fig 4-288). Bone-like hard tissue was visible at the alveolar crest and the lateral window area (black arrows on Figs 4-288c and d), and both implants attained good primary stability. Because an exposure of implant apex occurred at R1 (Fig 4-288f), autogenous bone chips were harvested from the same surgical field using EZ Bone Shaver (Pro-Seed, Japan) (blue arrow on Fig 4-288g) and placed over the exposed implant apex (yellow arrow on Fig 4-288h).

Second surgery was performed 6 months after the implant placement. Both of the implants achieved osseointegration (Figs 4-289 and 4-290). The superstructures were prepared by the patient's regular dentist. Postoperative follow-ups were performed in collaboration with the patient's regular dentist.

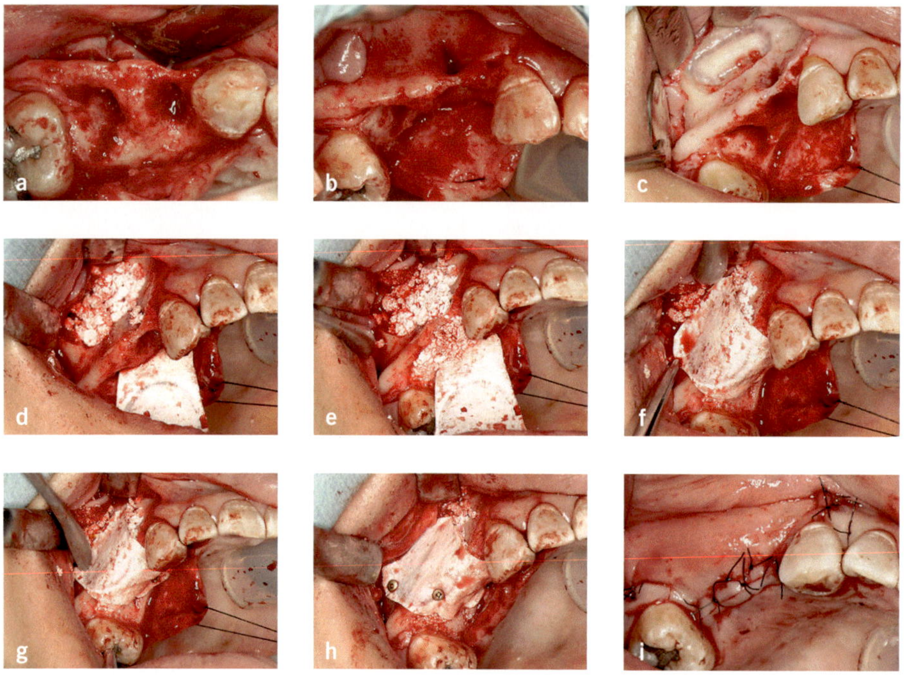

**Fig 4-287** (a to i) Intraoral views during the bone augmentation surgery.

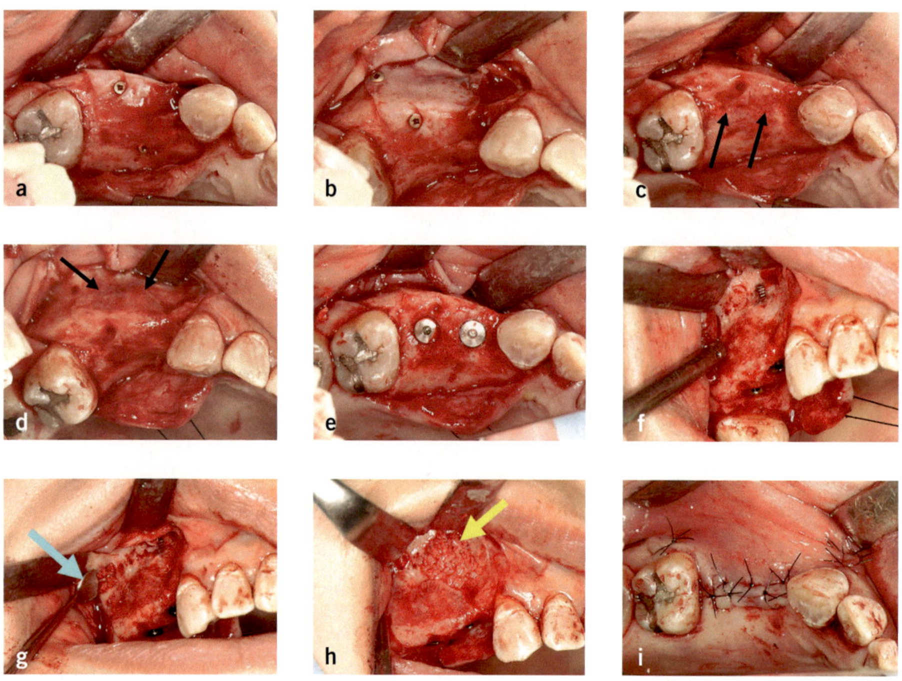

**Fig 4-288** (a to i) Intraoral views 1 year after the bone augmentation surgery.

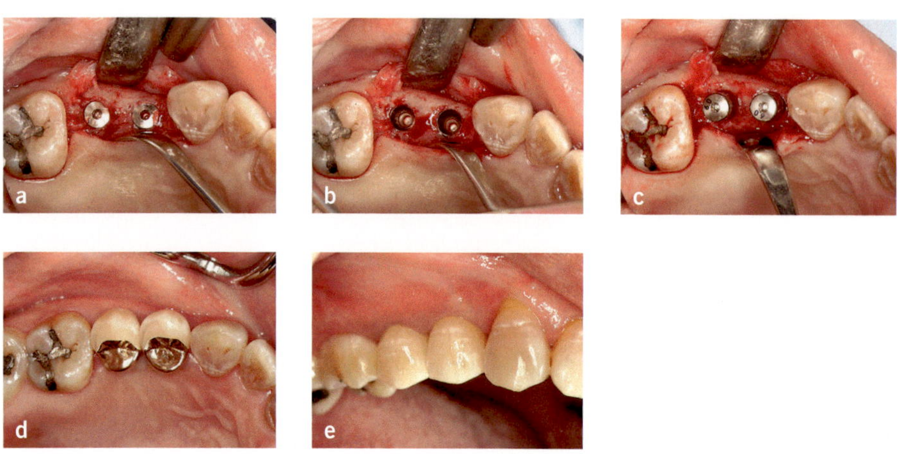

**Fig 4-289** (a to e) Intraoral views during the second surgery and after fabrication of superstructures.

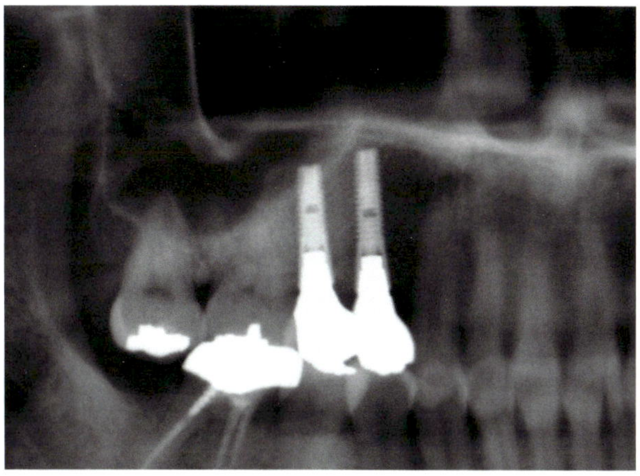

**Fig 4-290** Panoramic view after fabrication of superstructures.

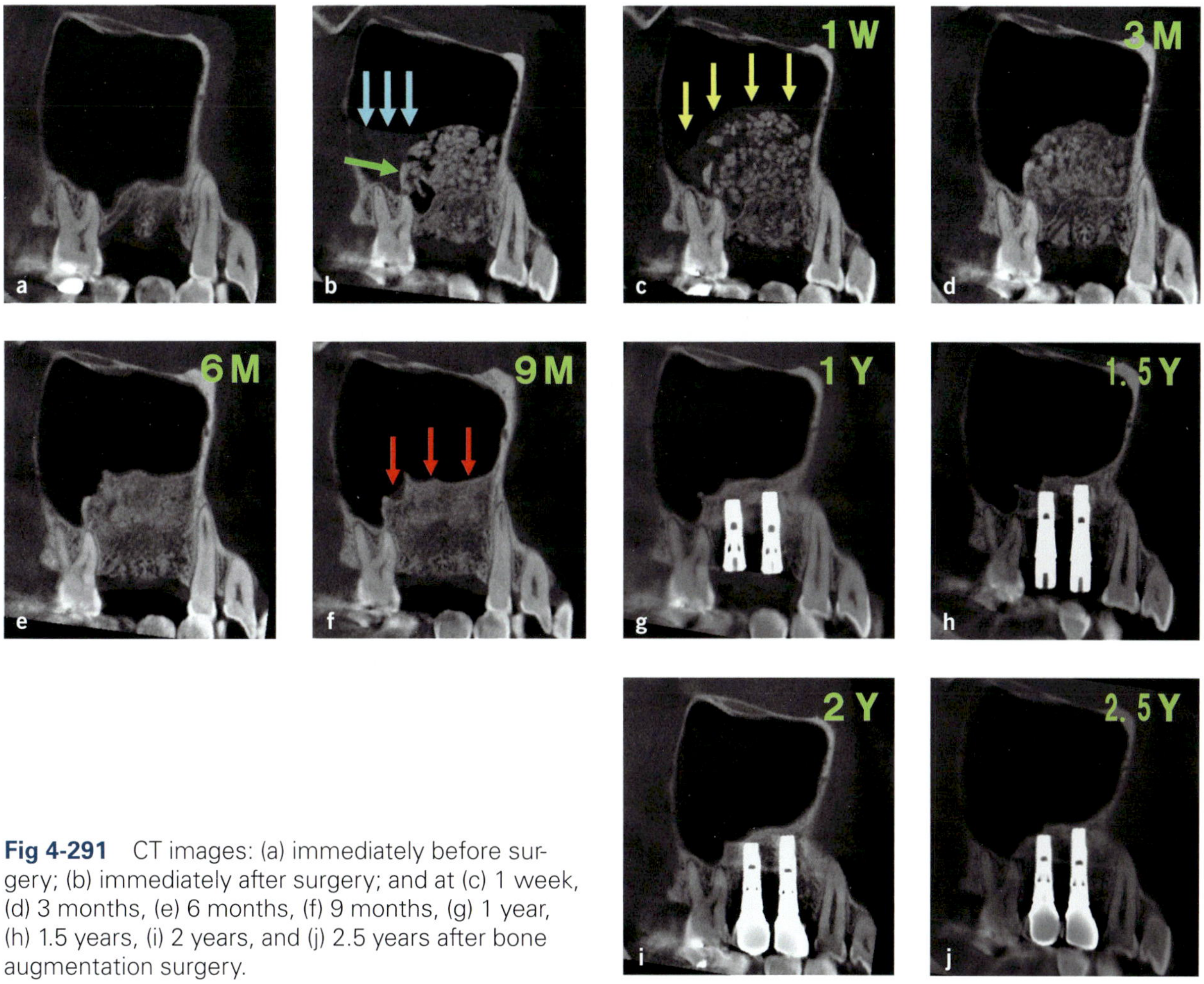


**Fig 4-291** CT images: (a) immediately before surgery; (b) immediately after surgery; and at (c) 1 week, (d) 3 months, (e) 6 months, (f) 9 months, (g) 1 year, (h) 1.5 years, (i) 2 years, and (j) 2.5 years after bone augmentation surgery.

Figure 4-291 shows a series of sagittal CT images obtained in the period from before surgery to 2.5 years after bone augmentation surgery. Because perforation of the maxillary sinus membrane occurred during sinus floor elevation, the bone at the lateral window was dissected and placed over the perforation (green arrow on Fig 4-291b). Therefore, retention of fluid, such as saline and blood within the maxillary sinus, was captured on the CT image taken immediately after surgery (blue arrows). One week afterwards, swelling occurred to the maxillary sinus membrane (yellow arrows on Fig 4-291c), which disappeared after 3 months. The sizes of individual β-TCP granules were reduced at the 3-month timepoint, and had become subtle by 6 months. Nine months after surgery, a cortical-bone–like radiopaque line was observed along the newly formed sinus floor (red arrows on Fig 4-291f), whereas the line of the original sinus floor looked blurred. Two years after surgery, cortical- and cancellous-bone–like radiopaque lines were observed at the augmented site, which was stable at 2.5 years after surgery.

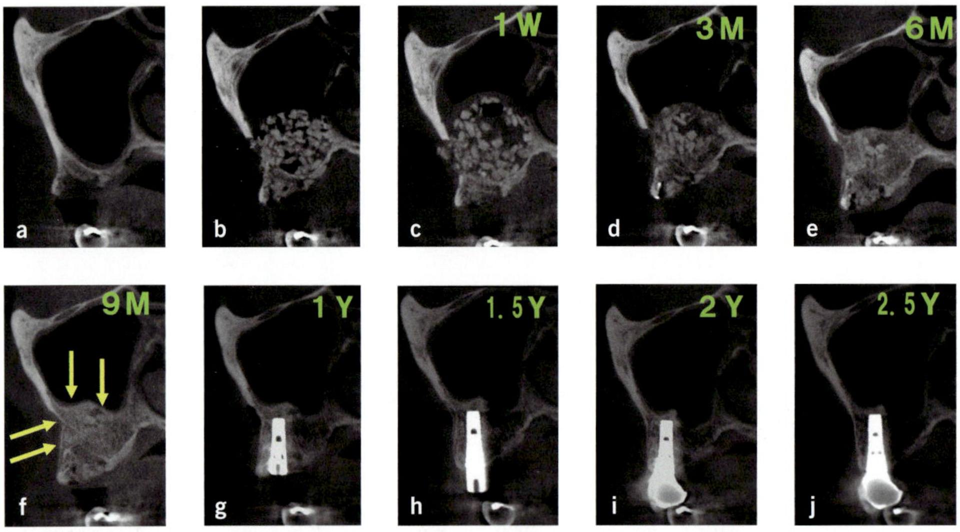


**Fig 4-292**
R2 region, buccolingual CT images: (a) immediately before surgery; (b) immediately after surgery; and at (c) 1 week, (d) 3 months, (e) 6 months, (f) 9 months, (g) 1 year, (h) 1.5 years, (i) 2 years, and (j) 2.5 years after surgery.

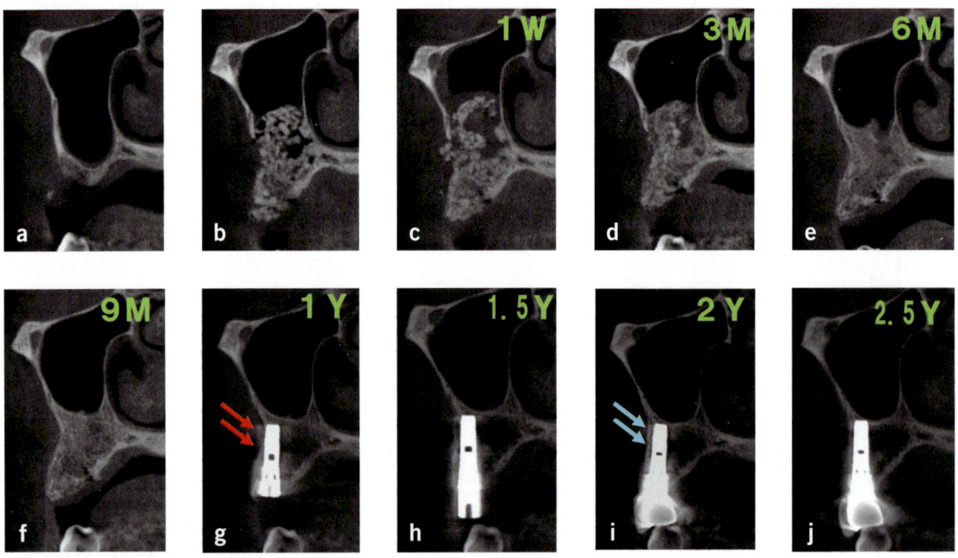


**Fig 4-293**
R1 region, buccolingual CT images: (a) immediately before surgery; (b) immediately after surgery; and at (c) 1 week, (d) 3 months, (e) 6 months, (f) 9 months, (g) 1 year, (h) 1.5 years, (i) 2 years, and (j) 2.5 years after surgery.

> **! Key Point**
>
> Two years after surgery, cortical- and cancellous-bone–like radiopaque lines were observed at the augmented site, which was stable at 2.5 years after surgery.

Figure 4-292 shows a series of buccolingual CT images at the R2 region. At 3 months after surgery, the size of β-TCP granules at the marginal area of the augmented site was reduced. Six months after surgery, the granules at the marginal area of the augmented site were even smaller but the granules at the center of the augmented area and GBR site maintained their original size and shape. Nine months after surgery, radiopaque lines were observed at the newly formed sinus floor and the lateral window area (yellow arrows on Fig 4-292f). Granules still remained at the center of the augmented region and GBR site but were now reduced in size. Two years after surgery, cortical and cancellous bone-like radiopacities were observed at the augmented site, which was stable at 2.5 years after surgery.

Figure 4-293 shows next a series of buccolingual CT images at the R1 region. Similar to the case of R2, the β-TCP granules began to gradually reduce in size, most strikingly at the marginal area and more subtly at the center. Moreover, the augmented site showed cortical-and cancellous-bone–like radiopacities. The autogenous bone chips employed during implant placement (red arrows on Fig 4-293g) changed over the course of the year to yield a cortical-bone–like dense radiopacity (blue arrows on Fig 4-293i).

> **! Key Point**
>
> The autogenous bone chips placed during implant placement (red arrows on Fig 4–293g) changed to give a cortical bone-like dense radiopacity over the course of 1 year (blue arrows on Fig 4-293i).

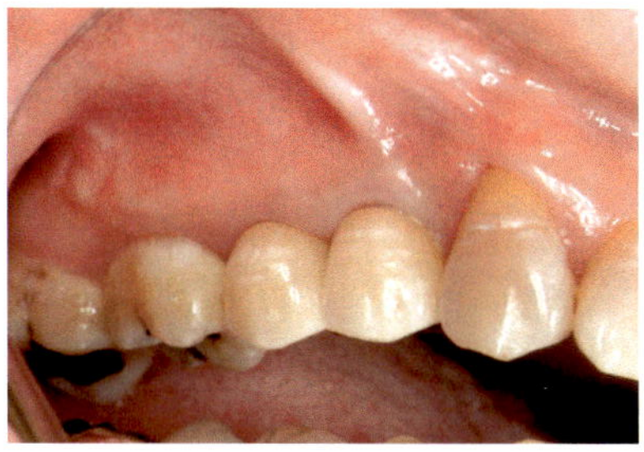

**Fig 4-294** (left) Intraoral view 3 years after surgery.

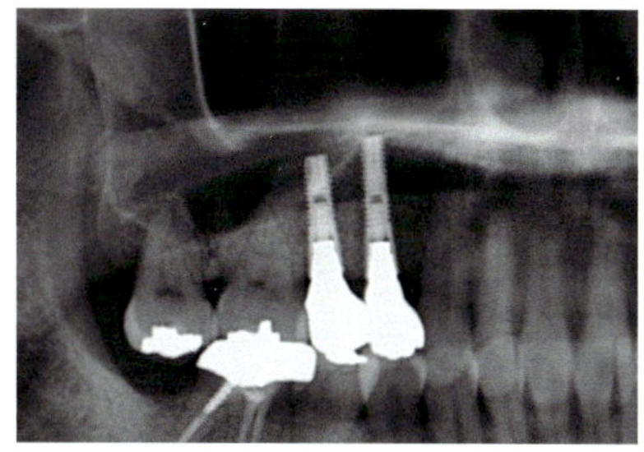

**Fig 4-295** (right) Panoramic view 3 years after surgery.

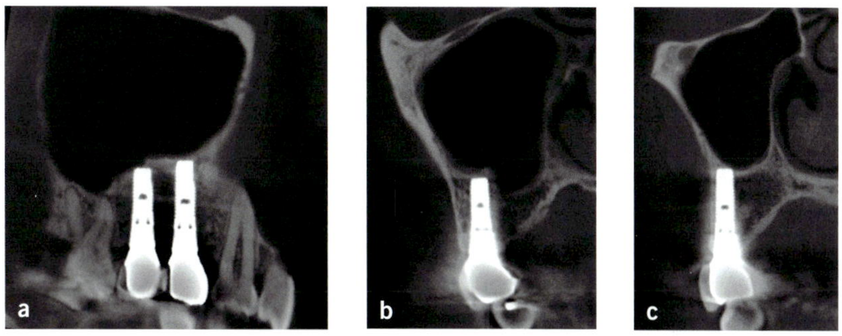

**Fig 4-296** (a to c) CT images 3 years after bone augmentation surgery.

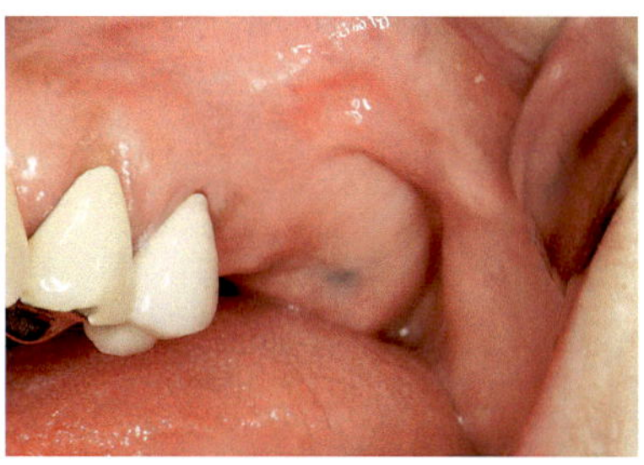

**Fig 4-297** Intraoral view at referral.

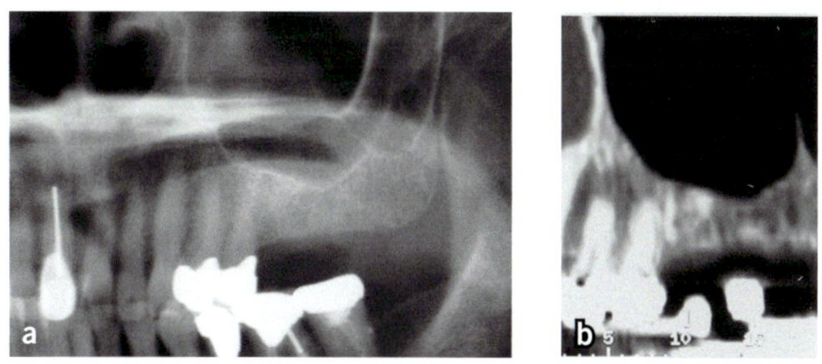

**Fig 4-298** (a and b) Panoramic views at eferral.

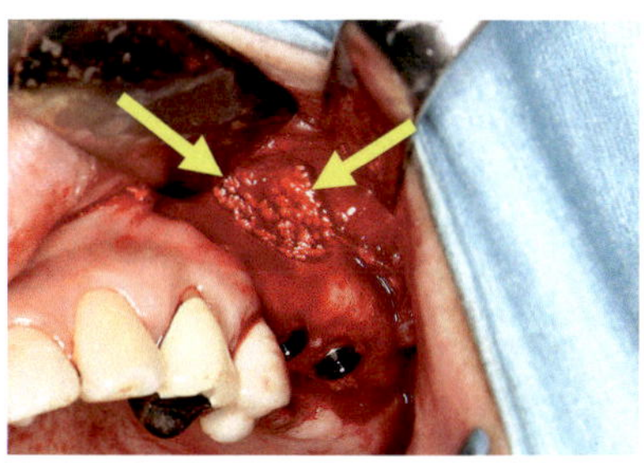

**Fig 4-299** (left) Intraoral view during bone augmentation surgery.

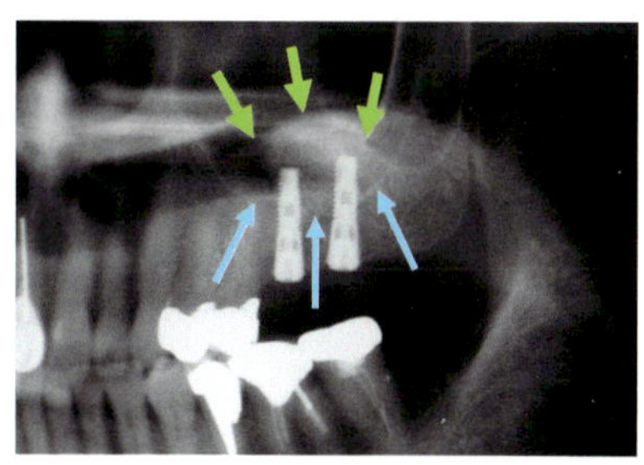

**Fig 4-300** (right) Panoramic view immediately after bone augmentation surgery.

Finally, images obtained 3 years after bone augmentation surgery are shown (Figs 4-294 to 4-296). There is no indication of peri-implant mucosal inflammation, and the prognosis is favorable. Although slight changes to the shape of the inferior concha can be seen on the CT image, the peri-implant bone looks identical to the way it did at 2.5 years. The β-TCP granules now show cortical- and cancellous-bone-like radiopacities, indicating that the active modeling and remodeling of the bone occurring after surgery has almost settled.

> **! Key Point**
>
> Active modeling and remodeling of the augmented bone appears to be settled at 3 years.

## Clinical report 11B: Sinus floor elevation using β-TCP alone

This patient with loss of teeth 26 and 27 was referred for implant placement. The residual bone heights at regions 26 and 27 were 7 mm and 5 mm, respectively (Figs 4-297 and 4-298). Implants were placed with simultaneous sinus floor elevation using β-TCP granules alone (Figs 4-299 and 4-300). After elevation of the maxillary sinus membrane, two implants were inserted and primary stability was achieved for both of them. The space around each implant was filled with β-TCP granules (yellow arrows on Fig 4-299).

Radiopacity of the augmented mass (green arrows on Fig 4-300) is shown on the panoramic radiograph taken immediately after surgery, and the

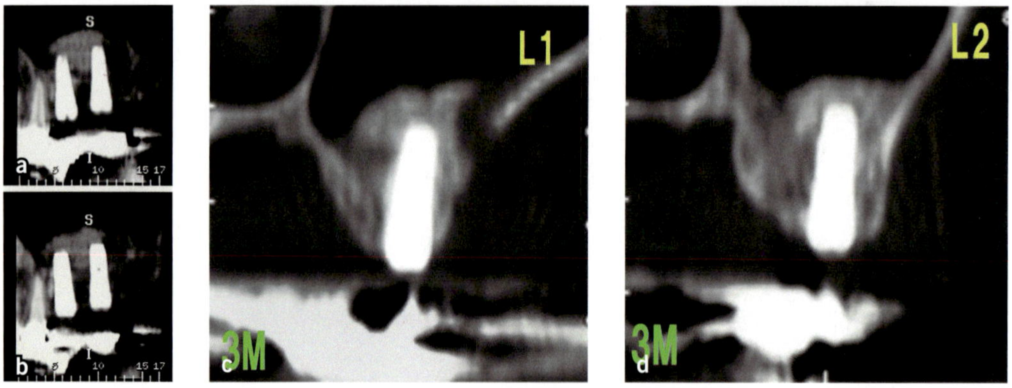


**Fig 4-301** (a to d) CT images 3 months after surgery.

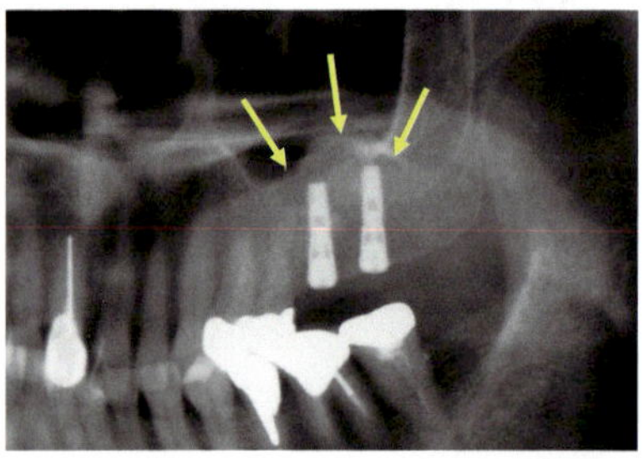

**Fig 4-302** (left) Panoramic view 1 year after surgery.

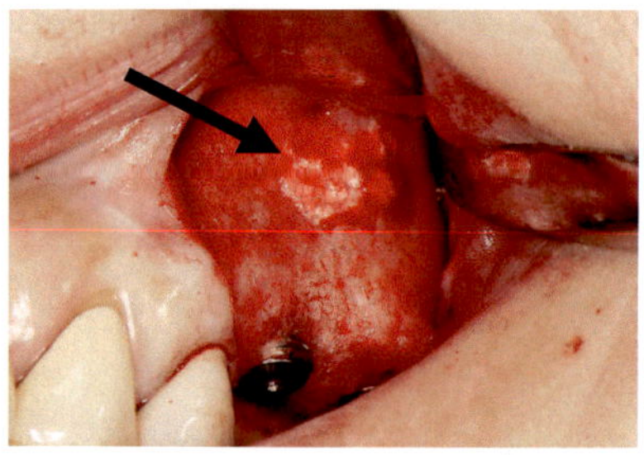

**Fig 4-303** (right) Intraoral image 1 year after surgery.

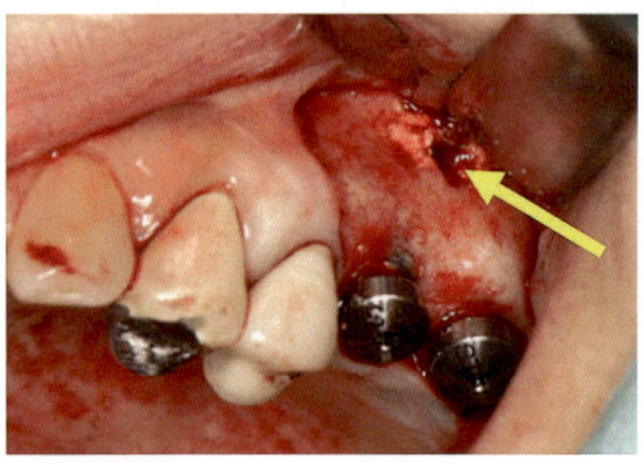

**Fig 4-304** Site of trephine bur biopsy.

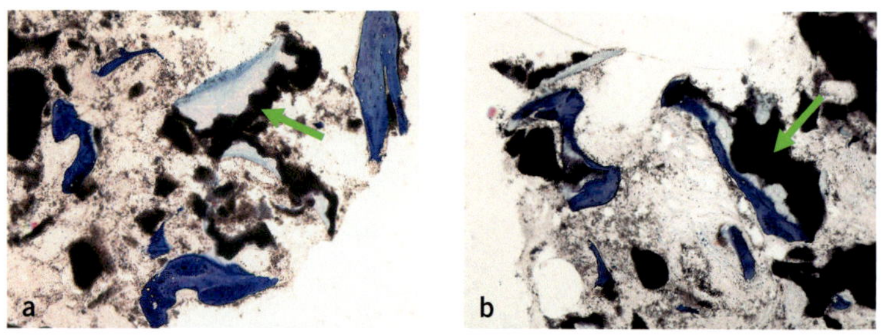


**Fig 4-305** (a and b) Histopathological sections stained with toluidine blue.

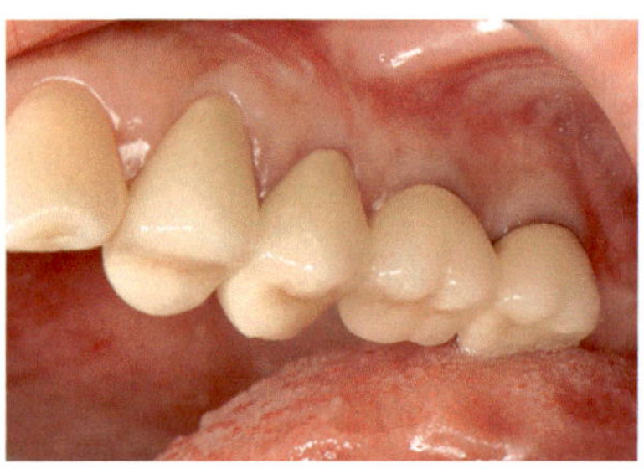

**Fig 4-306** (left) Absence of peri-implant gingival inflammation.

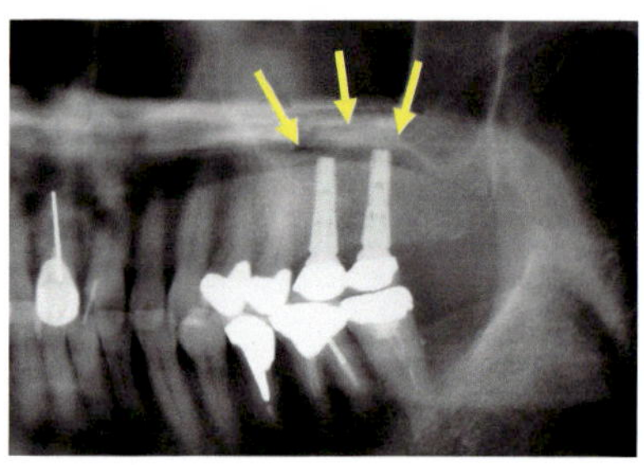

**Fig 4-307** (right) Panoramic view 1.5 years after sinus floor elevation.

line of the original sinus floor is also evident (blue arrows). While radiopacity around the implants can be seen on the helical CT image at 3 months, there is no sign of swelling of the maxillary sinus membrane (Fig 4-301).

On the panoramic radiograph 1 year after surgery, a radiopaque line was observed along the newly formed sinus floor (yellow arrows on Fig 4-302), whereas the line of the original sinus floor looked blurred. The β-TCP granules appeared to have been replaced with bone, and second surgery was performed. New bone was formed in the marginal area of the lateral window, but some residual granules were observed in the central area (black arrow on Fig 4-303).

With the patient's consent, trephine bur biopsy was performed at the center of the lateral window (yellow arrow on Fig 4-304), and histopathological sections were stained with toluidine blue (Fig 4-305). The residual β-TCP granules stained a dark brown color (green arrows on Fig 4-305a and b). Newly formed bone stained blue, and was observed around the residual granules. As seen on the image, new bone is formed gradationally from the surface of β-TCP granules.

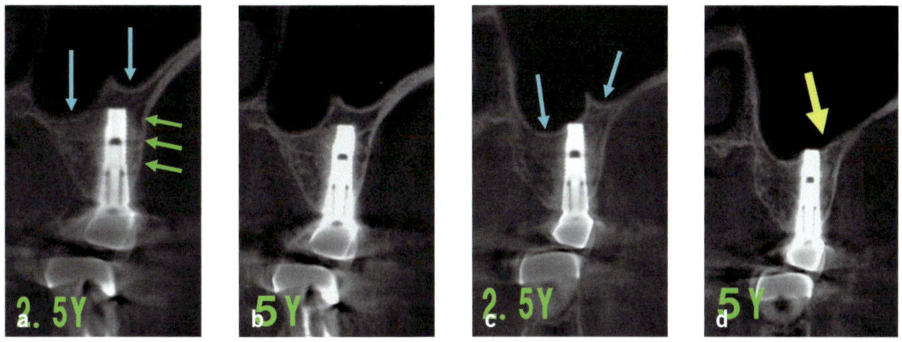


**Fig 4-308** (a and b) L1 at 2.5 and 5 years, respectively; (c and d) L2 at 2.5 and 5 years, respectively.

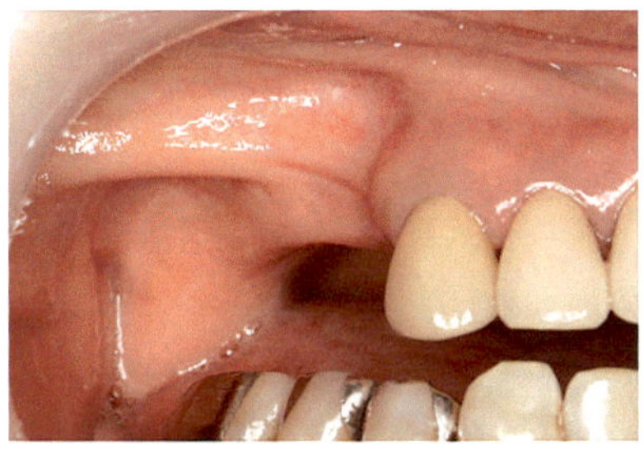

**Fig 4-309** (left) Intraoral view at referral.

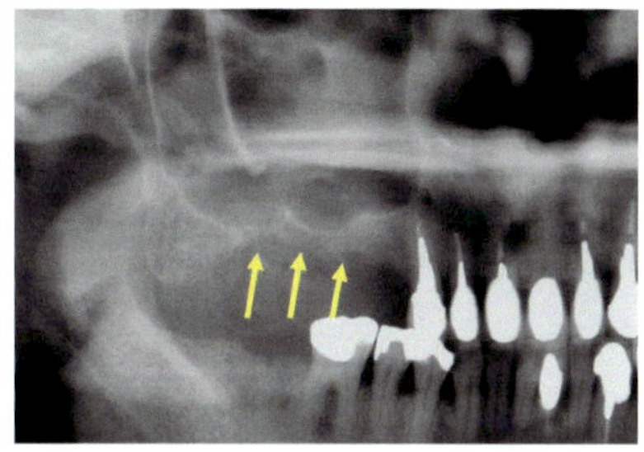

**Fig 4-310** (right) Panoramic view at referral.

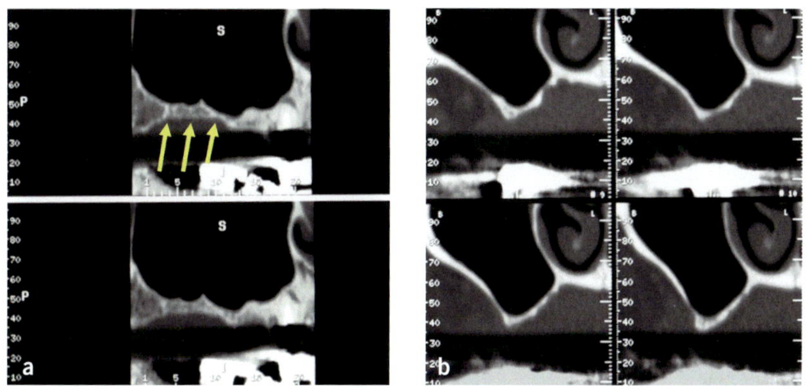


**Fig 4-311** (a and b) Helical CT images at referral.

The superstructures were prepared by the patient's regular dentist, and no sign of peri-implant gingival inflammation was detected (Fig 4-306). On a panoramic radiograph 1.5 years after sinus floor elevation, the radiopaque line of the original sinus floor had disappeared and a radiopaque line of the newly formed sinus floor was observed (yellow arrows on Fig 4-307).

Finally, buccolingual CT images were obtained at 2.5 years and 5 years after this surgery. At 2.5 years, cortical-bone–like radiopaque lines were observed at the lateral window area on the buccal aspect of L1 (green arrows on Fig 4-308a) and the newly formed sinus floor (blue arrows on Figs 4-408a and c). The radiopacities of the augmented area presented cortical- and cancellous-bone–like appearances. At 5 years, no changes to the augmented area were observed except for bone resorption on the sinus side of L2 (yellow arrow on Fig 4-308d).

> **! Key Point**
>
> On the buccolingual CT images 5 years after surgery, no changes to the augmented site were observed except for bone resorption on the sinus side of L2 (yellow arrow on Fig 4-308d).

## Clinical report 11C: Sinus floor elevation using β-TCP alone

This patient with loss of teeth 14–17 was referred for implant placement (Fig 4-309). A panoramic radiograph and helical CT indicated extensive development of the maxillary sinus and resorption of alveolar bone (yellow arrows on Figs 4-310 and 4-311).

In accordance with the patient's desire for sinus floor elevation using β-TCP, a sinus floor elevation procedure and simultaneous alveolar guided bone regeneration were performed under local anesthesia.

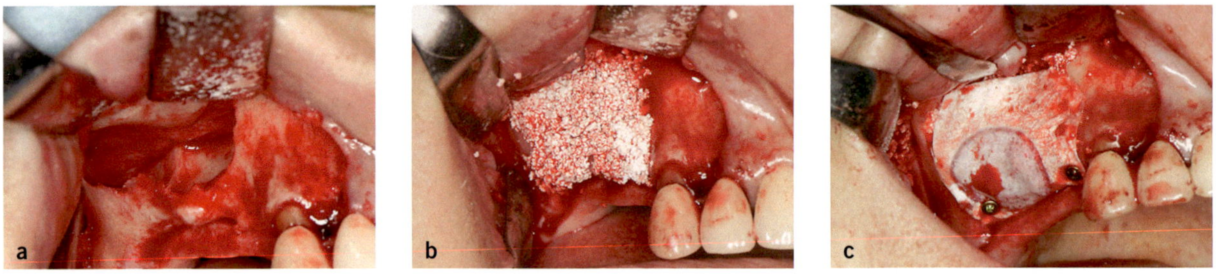

Fig 4-312 (a to c) Intraoperative intraoral views.

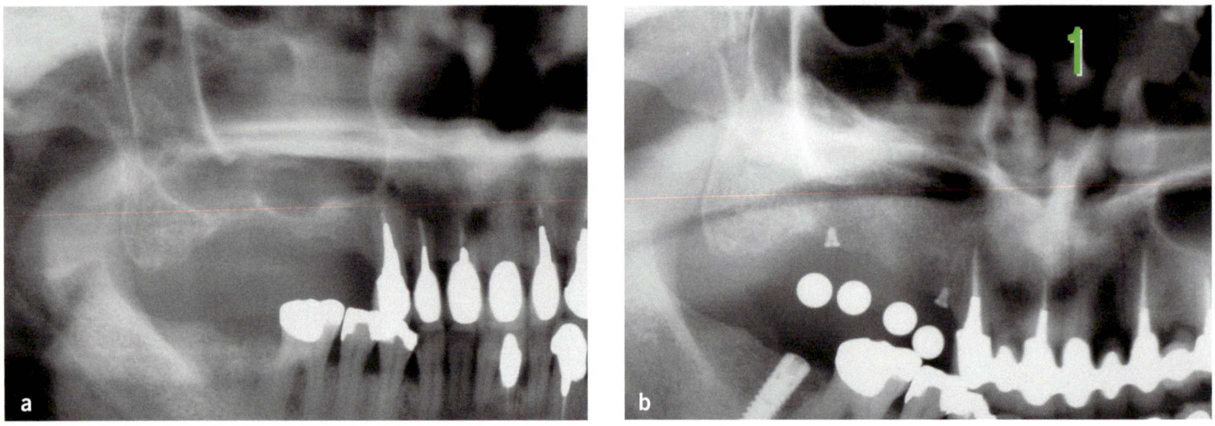

Fig 4-313 Panoramic views: (a) before, and (b) 1 year after surgery.

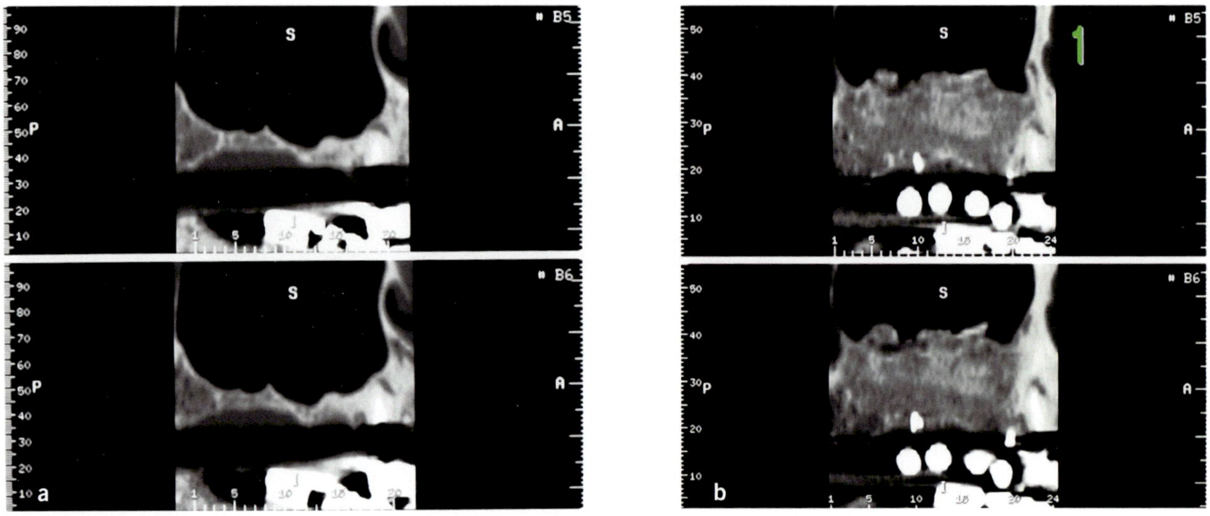

Fig 4-314 Helical CT images: (a) before, and (b) 1 year after surgery.

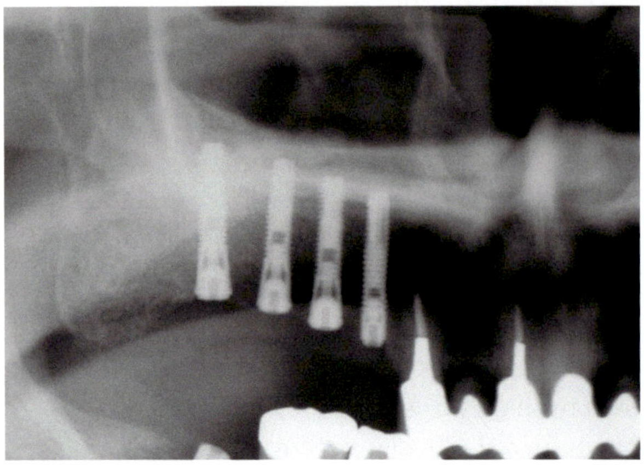

Fig 4-315 Panoramic view after the placement of implants.

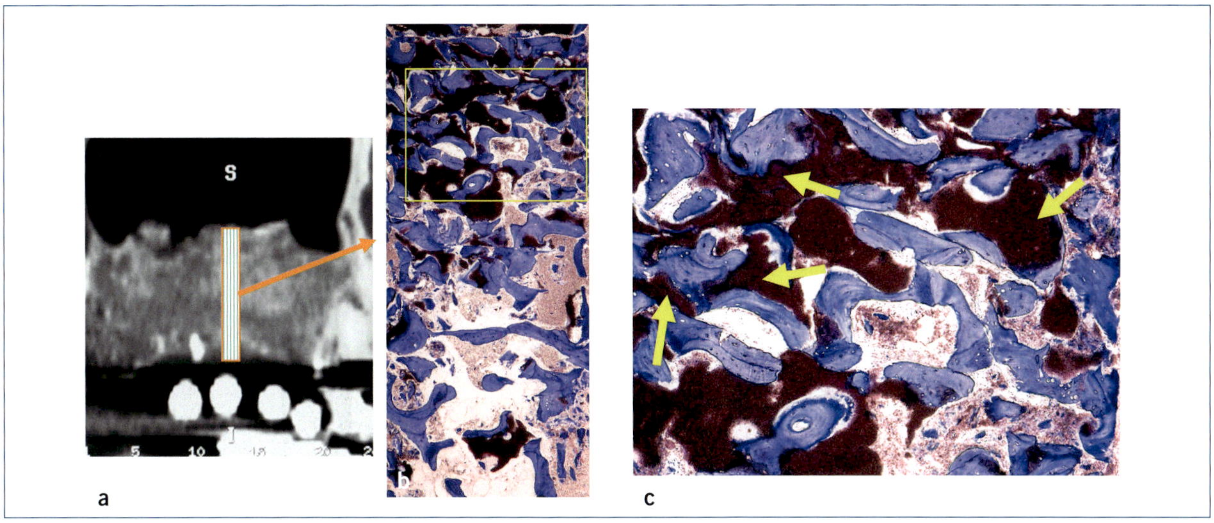


**Fig 4-316** (a to c) Histopathological analysis of the region of R3.

**Fig 4-317** (left) Intraoral view 4 years after surgery.

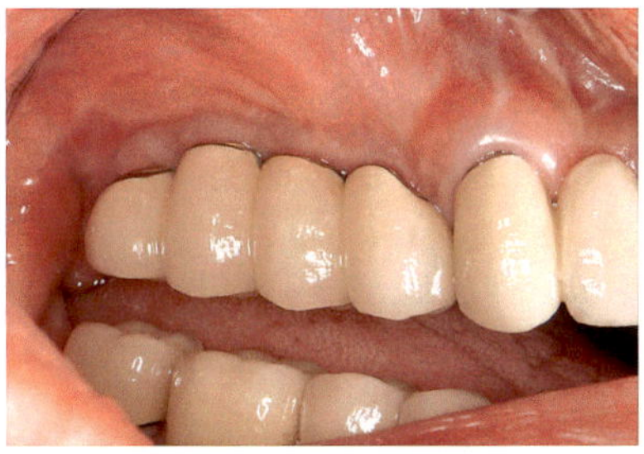

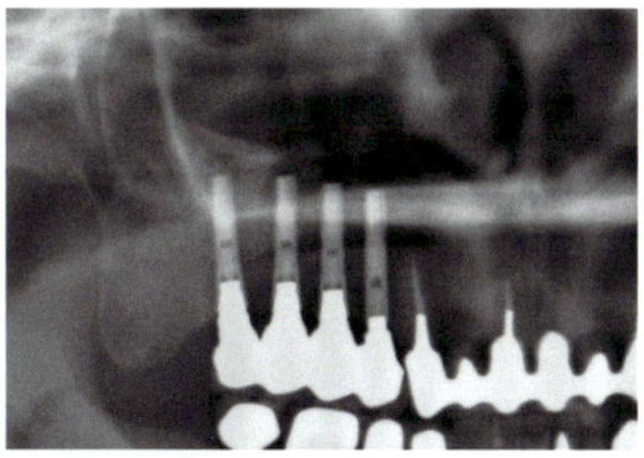

**Fig 4-318** (right) Panoramic view 4 years after surgery.

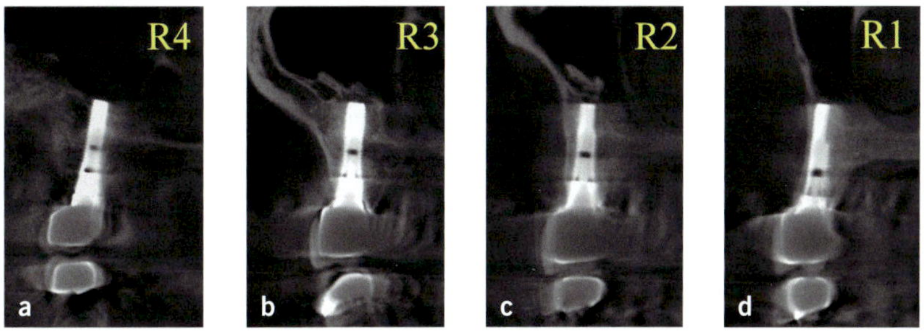


**Fig 4-319** (a to d) Buccolingual CT images 4 years after surgery.

After creation of the lateral window and elevation of the maxillary sinus membrane, β-TCP granules were inserted into the space created by the membrane elevation and placed over the alveolar crest as well (Figs 4-312a and b). The augmented site was then covered with a non-resorbable barrier membrane, and the wound was closed after making an appropriate release incision (Fig 4-312c).

Panoramic radiographs and helical CT images obtained 1 year after the surgery demonstrated radiopacities of the augmented site (Figs 4-313 and 4-314).

One year after sinus floor elevation, the non-resorbable barrier membrane was removed and four implants were placed (Fig 4-315). Trephine bur biopsy was performed at the region of R3.

Histopathological analysis of the region of R3 is shown in Figure 4-316. Newly formed bone can be seen at the R3 region, but some β-TCP granules still remained. The residual granules were incorporated into the newly formed bone (yellow arrows), demonstrating that residual β-TCP was being transformed into bone.

The augmented bone, however, was very soft to drill and did not seem to have mechanical strength to resist the occlusal load. After a 5-month healing period for the implants, the second surgery was performed and every implant had successfully osseointegrated. The superstructure was manufactured by the patient's regular dentist. Postoperative follow-up has been performed in collaboration with the patient's regular dentist.

Finally, images were obtained 4 years after the surgery (Figs 4-317 to 4-319). There was no evidence of peri-implant gingival inflammation and sufficient-

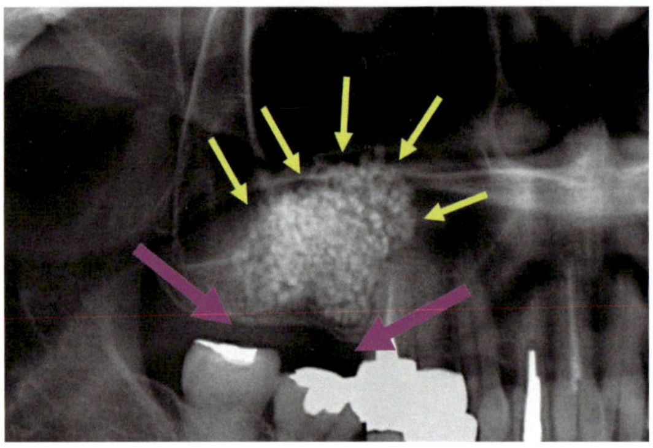

**Fig 4-320** Panoramic view on presentation.

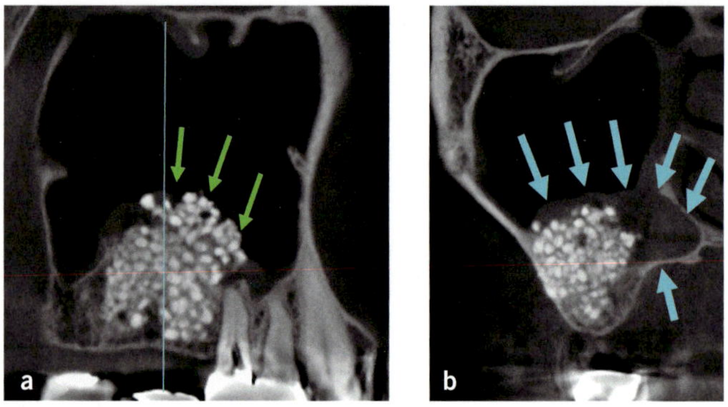


**Fig 4-321** (a and b) CT images on presentation.

ly dense radiopacity was observed around the implants. The radiopacities on the CT images indicated the formation of cortical- and cancellous-like bone.

**! Key Point**

The radiopacities on the CT images taken 4 years after surgery indicated the formation of cortical- and cancellous-like bone in the augmented region.

## Difficulty of evaluation of sinus floor elevation with non-resorbable bone substitutes

The author uses either β-TCP or autogenous bone (iliac bone marrow particulates) alone as the grafting material for sinus floor elevation. Because both materials form cortical- and cancellous-like bones through remodeling processes by about 2 years, it is easy to evaluate the newly formed bone tissue by CT scanning.

On the other hand, non-resorbable bone substitutes persist as a radiopaque substance and are said to be advantageous in preventing reduction of augmented volume. However, radiopacities do not always indicate bone tissue. Adequate mechanical strength of the augmented mass cannot be achieved until the new bone formed around the bone substitute granules have fused. Therefore, CT evaluation of the postoperative situation of non-resorbable bone substitutes is difficult.

**! Key Point**

It should be noted that radiopacities of bone substitute granules cannot be taken as bone tissue.

### Clinical report 12: Two-year follow-up of sinus floor elevation with non-resorbable bone substitutes

This patient received sinus floor elevation at another clinic 2 years earlier and was referred on by a different dentist. A panoramic radiograph showed granular-shaped radiopacities in the augmented region (yellow arrows on Fig 4-320). However, the clearances at regions 16 and 17 were too small to support superstructures (pink arrows).

On our CT images, the outer shape of the substitute mass was clearly observed with some loose granules in the upper layer of the augmented area (green arrows on Fig 4-321a). In contrast, mild swelling of the maxillary sinus membrane was observed around the bone substitutes (blue arrows on Fig 4-321b), indicative of minor inflammation.

With non-resorbable bone substitutes, the granules function as the core over which new bone is formed. When the new bone formed around the granules fuses with each other, the augmented area can gain mechanical strength. In this patient it was unclear, despite 2 years of healing, whether bone had been formed around the bone substitutes, and implant placement was considered to pose a risk of implant failure. Owing to their radiopacity, non-resorbable bone substitute materials are thought to be useful as filling material. However, the mechanical strength of non-resorbable bone substitutes placed in the augmented region cannot be assessed, even by CT scans. Furthermore, there exists the possibility of providing misleading information pertaining to bone density (eg, grossly overestimating bone density) if evaluated only by the CT values (Hounsfield values).

Conversely, with autogenous bone grafts and resorbable bone substitutes (such as β-TCP), modeling and remodeling of these materials can be evaluated by CT. Therefore, the author believes that autogenous bone grafts and resorbable bone substitutes are a better choice of filling materials for sinus floor elevation.

**! Key Point**

Even 2 years following surgery, non-resorbable bone substitutes manifest radiopacity. However, whether new bone has been formed around the granules remains unclear, and some loose granules are observed in the upper area of the augmented mass. Therefore, the mechanical strength of the augmented bone is questionable, leading to a concern about implant stability.

# PART 2 The osteotome technique aided by CT scanning

# CHAPTER 5

# Principles and procedures of the osteotome technique

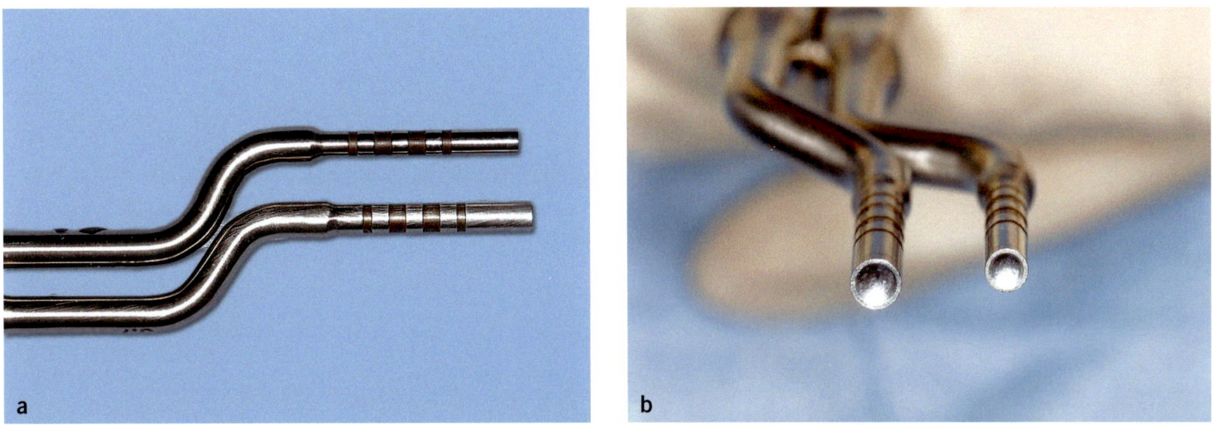

Fig 5-1 (a and b) Examples of the instruments used for the osteotome technique.

## Introduction

The osteotome technique is applicable in cases with a residual bone height of 6–8 mm to the maxillary sinus membrane. It facilitates implant placement by elevating the maxillary sinus floor using a crestal approach. Because this sinus floor elevation uses a set of special instruments called osteotomes, it is referred to as the osteotome technique, or osteotome sinus floor elevation (OSFE) (Fig 5-1).

It is growing in popularity because it is less invasive and seems to be simpler to perform than sinus floor elevation by the lateral window technique. However, it should be noted that there are some drawbacks to this procedure.

## Basics of the surgical procedure

1. Drill the implant socket from the ridge crest, leaving the cortical bone plate (1–2 mm) of the maxillary sinus floor intact (Fig 5-2).
2. Insert a special osteotome into the implant socket through the ridge crest and gently and carefully tap the cortical plate at the bottom of the sinus to fracture superiorly (Fig 5-3).
3. Using an instrument such as a depth gauge inserted through the ridge crest, push up the sinus membrane around the fractured cortical plate.
4. Check for membrane perforation by applying positive pressure inside the oral cavity (instruct patients to balloon their cheeks) and check whether air leaks through the nostrils.
5. Insert a depth gauge and determine the length within the range where the fractured bone plate is pushed back with the elasticity of the sinus membrane. Insert the implant.

The level of difficulty of sinus membrane elevation varies from patient to patient. In particular, membrane elevation at the medial site of the sinus cavity is often challenging (green arrow on Fig 5-3).

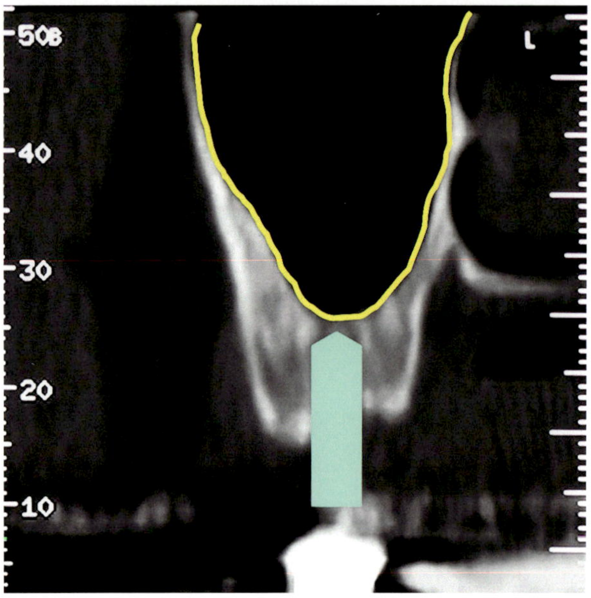


**Fig 5-2** Drilling the implant socket.

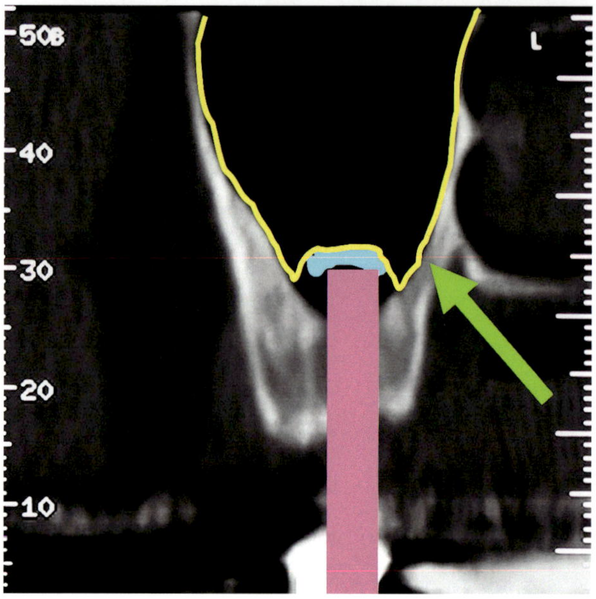


**Fig 5-3** Tapping the cortical plate gently.

> **! Key Point**
>
> The method of inducing positive pressure inside the sinus cavity by pinching the nostrils and checking whether air flows into the oral cavity is unreliable, because a torn membrane may work as a valve to prevent the air from leaking.

## Advantages and disadvantages

### Advantages

Compared with sinus floor elevation by the lateral window technique, this:

- is less invasive
- seems to be simpler.

### Disadvantages

1. Because the osteotome technique is an invisible procedure, pre- and postoperative evaluation is impossible without CT.
2. Because a membrane perforation, should it occur, makes the osteotome technique impossible, surgical reliability is lower.
3. Inadequate volume of bone substitute granules or autogenous bone particulates may cause membrane perforation and lead to maxillary sinusitis.
4. An implant placed with the osteotome technique may not achieve osseointegration if primary implant stability cannot be attained due to reduced residual bone volume.
5. An implant may fall into the sinus cavity if primary implant stability cannot be attained and there is membrane perforation.
6. The implant length that can be placed is limited, and there is concern about the long-term prognosis of shorter implants.
7. Complications, if they occur, will require more invasive recovery procedures than the original surgery, which leads to loss of the patient's trust.

## Discussion

The author views the osteotome technique as a sinus floor elevation procedure associated with high risk. In recent years it has been gaining popularity with its suggested decreased invasiveness. However, it should be noted that complications associated with the osteotome technique have also been sharply increasing. In particular, the credibility of clinical cases reported without providing postoperative CT evidence is questionable and it is too risky to regard them as clinically successful cases.

# CHAPTER 6

# Pitfalls of the osteotome technique

## Informed consent

The osteotome technique is becoming common as a less invasive method for sinus floor elevation. However, it has the drawback of being invisible surgery. It also carries risks, including:

- premature discontinuation of the surgery
- perforation of the sinus membrane
- dislocation of the implant into the sinus cavity
- complications such as postoperative infection.

The author believes that this technique is more difficult than the lateral window technique because it is invisible surgery. If we recommend the osteotome technique to our patients using "less invasive" as the key phrase, we may face difficulties in the future because postoperative complications, if they occur, require more invasive treatment than the original osteotome technique itself.

### Suggested explanation of the risks to the patient

- If the sinus membrane becomes perforated, implant placement becomes impossible and premature discontinuation of surgery is unavoidable.
- At least 6 months will be necessary before adequate new bone regeneration at the osteotomy site and healing of perforated membrane occurs.
- After the aforementioned healing, sinus floor elevation using the lateral window technique and bone substitutes is necessary for implant placement. Even if the implant is placed simultaneously with the sinus floor elevation, a healing period of about a year is necessary before the second surgery.
- If the osteotome technique fails, the entire treatment period will be delayed by 6 months, compared with a case where the patient is treated from the start with sinus floor elevation by the lateral window technique.

> **! Key Point**
>
> It is of extreme importance to provide patients with in-depth detailed information on the procedure and any possible drawbacks or setbacks.

## Some clinical case reports

### Clinical report 1: A case with favorable prognosis after the osteotome technique

When sinus floor elevation is necessary, the author makes it a rule to explain to the patient the differences between the osteotome and lateral window techniques. By providing the patient with a good understanding of the advantages and disadvantages of both techniques, the author makes the patient choose the technique for sinus augmentation.

> **! Key Point**
>
> It is crucial to explain the recovery plan to the patient, in case the osteotome technique results in failure.

In this patient, the residual bone height to the sinus floor was about 6 mm and both techniques were viable treatment options (Fig 6-1). When thinking of the implant insertion direction, it was determined possible to fracture the sinus floor perpendicularly to the tangential direction of the maxillary sinus floor (blue line on Fig 6-1b). Based on the treatment plan, explained in detail, the patient chose the osteotome technique.

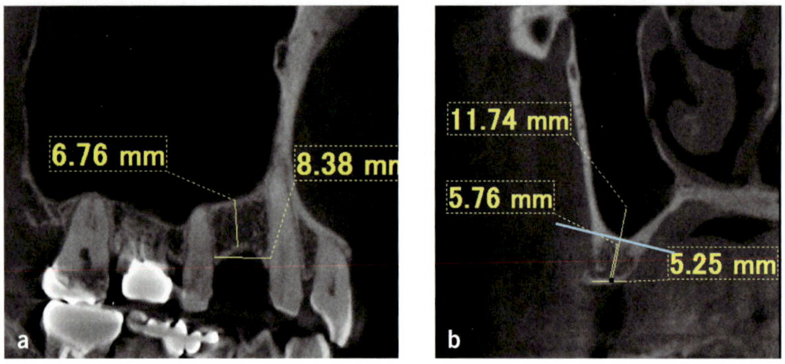


**Fig 6-1** (a and b) Preoperative assessment CT images.

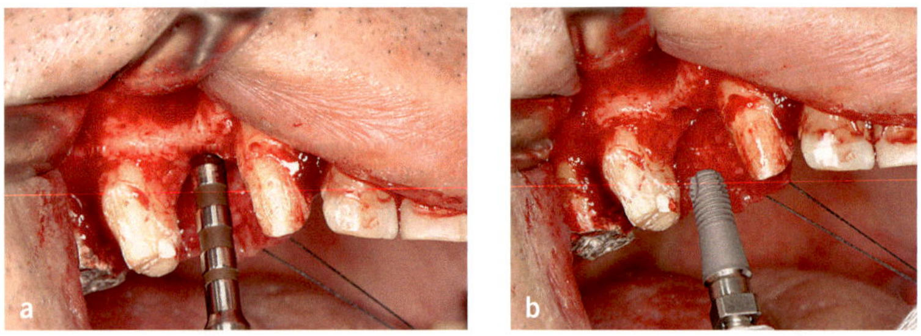


**Fig 6-2** (a and b) Osteotome technique for the 11 mm implant.

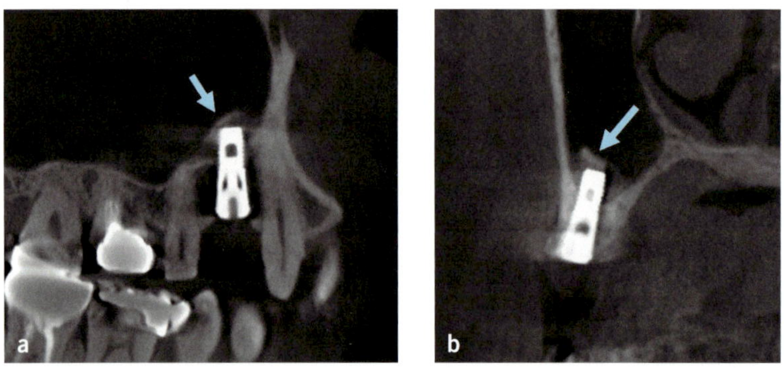


**Fig 6-3** (a and b) CT images immediately after the surgery.

**! Key Point**

Elevate the sinus membrane while preventing perforation.

After drilling to a depth of about 5 mm, the cortical bone of the sinus floor was fractured using a set of osteotomes (Fig 6-2; see also Figs 5-1 to 5-3 in Chapter 5). Because the fractured bone plate could be elevated without causing any perforation to the membrane, an 11 mm implant was inserted and good primary stability could be achieved.

**! Key Point**

Procedures to fill the space created by the osteotome technique with grafting materials, such as bone substitutes and autogenous bone particulates, have often been reported. However, the process of space filling is invisible and membrane perforation caused by grafting materials, if it occurs, can be detected only by postoperative CT scanning.

Figure 6-3 shows CT images obtained immediately after the surgery. The radiopacities of the fractured bone plates can be seen on the implant apex (blue arrows). The elevated sinus membrane appears as a fan-shaped radiopacity with the bone plate at the top.

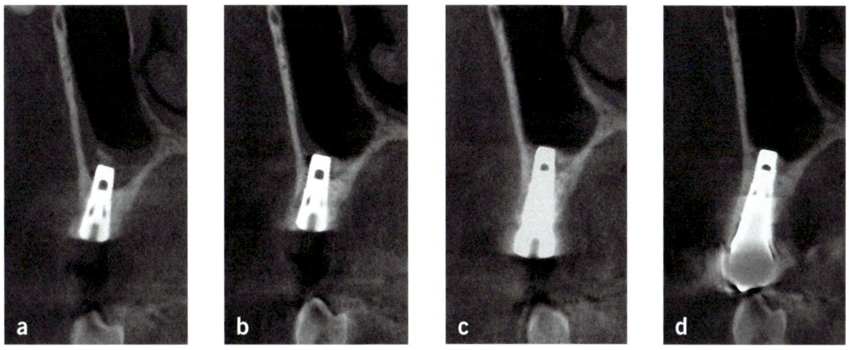


**Fig 6-4** CT images after surgery: (a) at 1 week; (b) at 3 months; (c) at 6 months; (d) at 1.5 years.

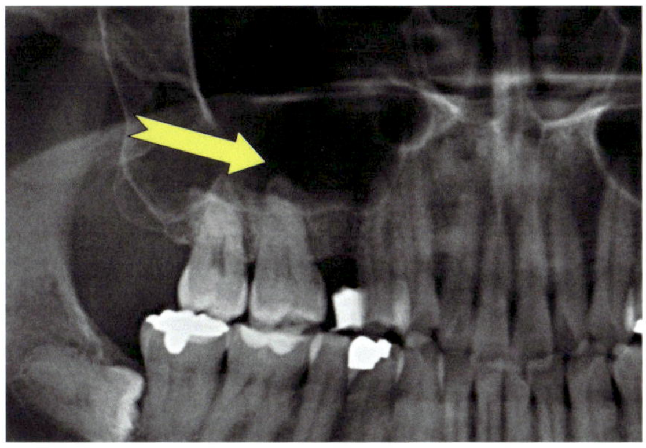

**Fig 6-5** (left) Panoramic view before surgery.

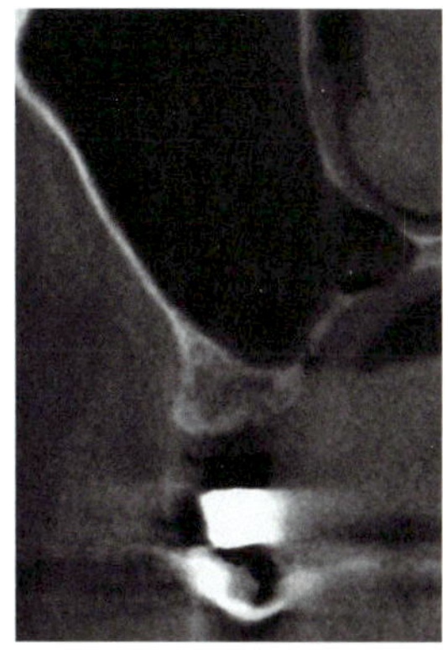

**Fig 6-6** (right) CT image before surgery.

> **! Key Point**
>
> Any damage to the sinus membrane results in failure of the osteotome technique and may lead to the onset of maxillary sinusitis. Therefore, the author does not use grafting material in the osteotome technique.

Figure 6-4 shows a series of postoperative buccolingual CT images. At 1 week there was membrane swelling. At 3 months, the swelling had lessened and the fractured bone plates had disappeared. At 6 months, the membrane swelling had completely dissipated and the radiopacity of the augmented area had become denser. On the image 1.5 years after surgery, the augmented site shows uniform radiopacity but the border of the native bone still remains unchanged.

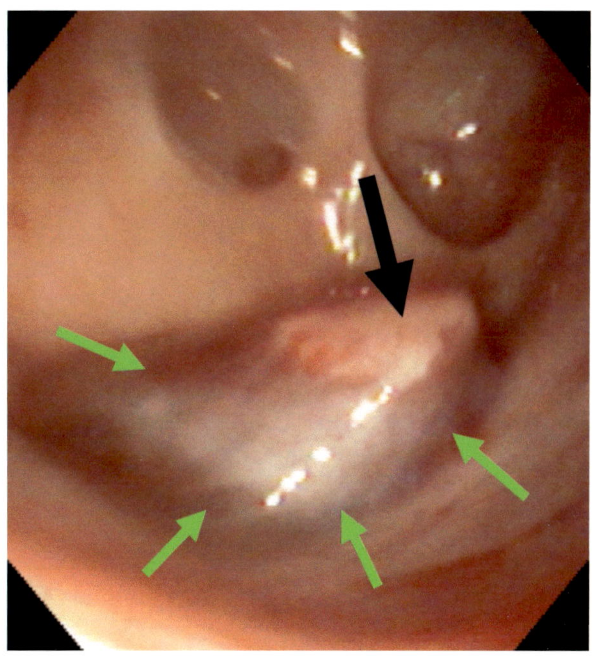

**Fig 6-7** View through the fiberscope.

## Clinical report 2: A case with uncertain prognosis after the osteotome technique

This patient had lost tooth 15 and desired implant treatment. The patient was a dentist with a full understanding of the risks associated with the osteotome technique. Nevertheless, though the residual bone height was 4–5 mm, he wanted sinus augmentation by the osteotome technique.

The surgery was performed (Figs 6-5 to 6-7). The condition of the sinus membrane was monitored with a fiberscope inserted through a hole drilled on the anterior wall of the sinus (yellow arrow on Fig 6-5), and an 11 mm implant was placed. The elevated bone plate (black arrow on Fig 6-7) and sinus membrane could be monitored by the fiberscope

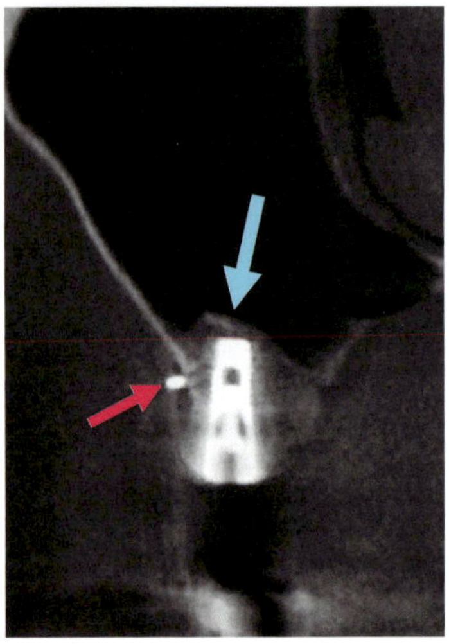

Fig 6-8 CT image immediately after surgery.

during the surgery, and accumulation of dark purple-colored blood was also found immediately beneath the sinus membrane (green arrows).

The implant attained good primary stability. In addition to the elevated bone plate (blue arrow on Fig 6-8), a fan-shaped radiopacity was observed at the augmented area on the buccolingual CT image taken immediately after surgery. The cross-section of the drain was also observed as a radiopacity on the buccal site of the alveolar ridge (red arrow on Fig 6-8).

Figure 6-9 shows postoperative buccolingual CT images. At 1 month, the swelling of the sinus membrane remained to some extent and the elevated bone plate had disappeared. Second surgery was performed 5 months after the implant placement, at which time there was no membrane swelling and radiopacities were observed at the augmented area. One year after surgery, the radiopacities at the augmented site were denser and the newly formed sinus floor was observed as a radiopaque line (yellow arrow on Fig 6-9c).

Although it appeared that the implant apex was protruding into the sinus cavity on the panoramic radiograph 2 years after surgery (Fig 6-10), no swelling was observed on the CT image and progress was considered satisfactory. However, the slight decrease of the bone level on the palatal side of the implant (pink arrow on Fig 6-9d) hinted at concerns about the long-term prognosis of the implant.

**! Key Point**

Reduction of bone level is a sign of an unfavorable prognosis.

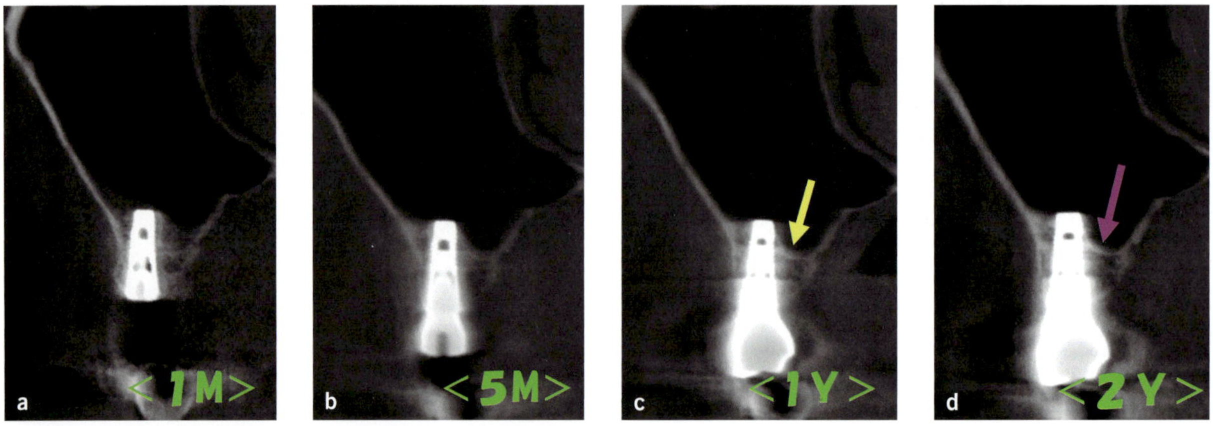


Fig 6-9 CT images after surgery: (a) at 1 month; (b) at 5 months; (c) at 1 year; (d) at 2 years.

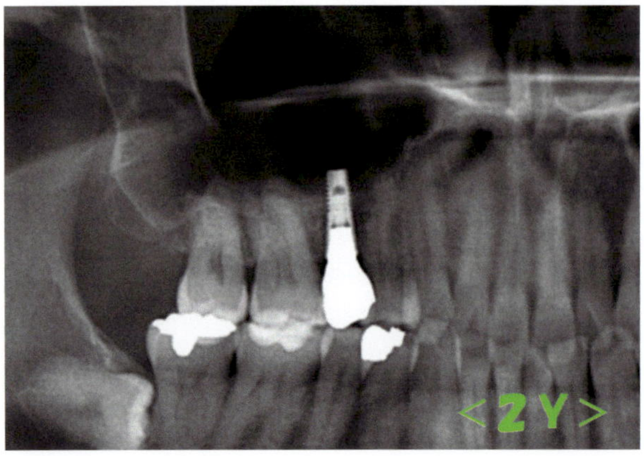


Fig 6-10 Panoramic view 2 years after surgery.

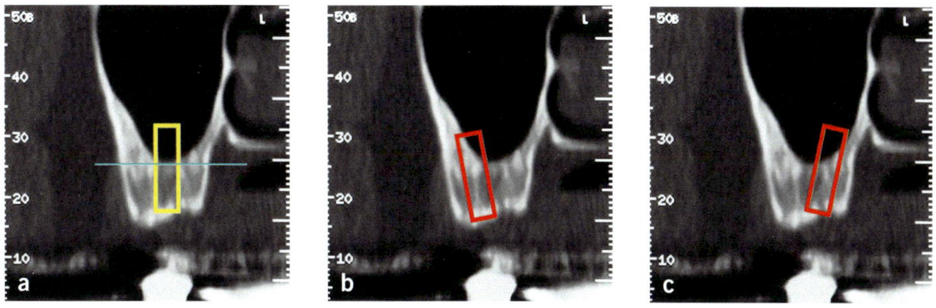


**Fig 6-11** (a to c) Three examples of insertion direction.

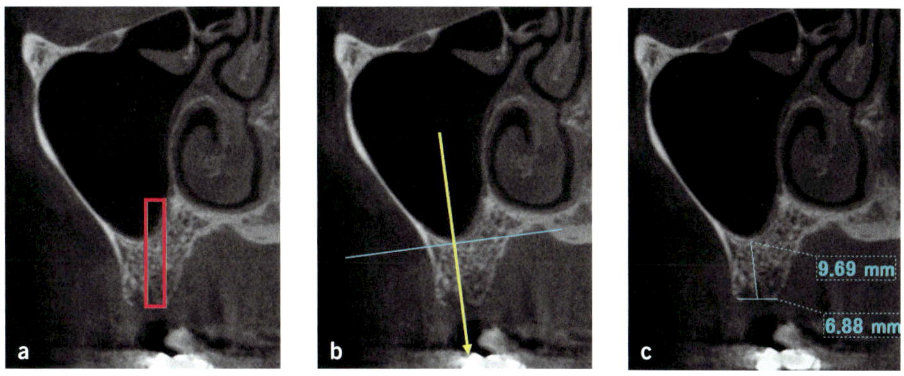


**Fig 6-12** (a to c) Preoperative CT imaging and assessment.

## Significance of the implant insertion direction

Sinus floor fracture perpendicular to the tangential line of the sinus floor is the commonly accepted approach of the osteotome technique. When an implant is inserted in the direction shown on Fig 6-11a, the osteotome technique is performed perpendicular to the tangential line of the sinus floor and the fracture of the bone plate is easy. In the situations shown in Figs 6-11b and 6-11c, however, sinus floor fracture is difficult and, even if fractured, there is a risk of sinus membrane perforation caused by applying excessive force. Therefore, preoperative examination by CT scanning is indispensable with the osteotome technique. Expertise in three-dimensional implant placement assessment is also required.

### Clinical report 3: Fracture of the sinus floor on the palatal aspect

When placing an implant as shown in Fig 6-12a, fracture of the sinus floor on the palatal aspect is considered difficult. However, if we follow the line that connects the ridge crest and the functional cusp of the antagonist and which is perpendicular to the tangential line of the sinus floor (blue line on Fig 6-12b), the implant is placed in the direction of the yellow arrow. In addition, the residual bone in the planned insertion direction has a height of 9.6 mm (Fig 6-12c), so at least a 9 mm implant can be placed. Based on the reasoning above, the osteotome technique was chosen in this case.

> **! Key Point**
>
> When choosing the osteotome technique, various requirements, including the residual bone volume, the sinus floor morphology and the implant insertion direction, have to be met. Preoperative evaluation by CT scan is indispensable, and the skills of defining three-dimensionally optimal insertion direction and accurate drilling technique are demanded.

During the surgery, it was determined that a 13 mm implant could be placed and good primary stability was achieved. The fractured bone plate was observed above the implant apex on the CT image taken immediately after surgery (yellow arrow on Fig 6-13a).

The second surgery was performed 5 months after the implant placement. The radiopacity of the augmented site was denser but some resorption was observed on the buccal alveolar bone (Fig 6-13b). One year after the implant placement, the radiopacity of the augmented site showed further increase

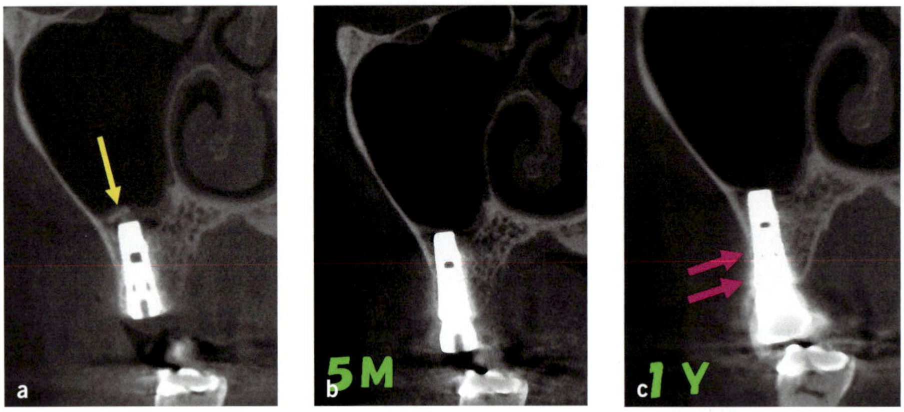


**Fig 6-13** CT images: (a) immediately after surgery; (b) at 5 months; (c) at 1 year.

in density, but the prognosis of the buccal bone level was still of concern (red arrows on Fig 6-13c).

## Misidentifying the sinus floor

Preoperative evaluation based solely on panoramic radiography is dangerous. If the nasal cavity is wide, the nasal cavity floor may produce a radiopaque line at the molar region and may be incorrectly diagnosed as the sinus floor. Assessing the insertion direction 3-dimensionally is important when using the osteotome technique, so CT scanning is indispensable.

### Clinical report 4: Nasal cavity floor misidentified

For a patient whose panoramic radiograph showed a clear radiopaque line in the upper area of the alveolar ridge, a CT scan was performed to check whether the osteotome technique procedure at the planned implant site (yellow squares on Fig 6-14a) was feasible. The CT image revealed that the radiopaque line on the panoramic radiograph, which had been interpreted as the sinus floor, was in fact the line of nasal cavity floor (the true sinus floor was the line shown by the green arrow on Figs 6-14a and b). If the diagnosis had been made based solely on the panoramic radiography, osteotome technique surgery might have been performed on the nasal cavity.

> **! Key Point**
>
> Diagnosis based solely on panoramic radiography is associated with a risk of performing osteotome technique surgery on the nasal cavity.

## Displacement of implant into the maxillary sinus

One of the most serious potential complications of the osteotome technique is displacement of the implant into the maxillary sinus. In recent years, some have said that the osteotome technique is applicable to residual bone with a height of only several millimeters, but the author believes that to be extremely dangerous.

The recovery procedure for an implant displaced into the maxillary sinus is far more invasive than the osteotome technique itself and will cause significant morbidity for the patient. Further, if the patient sees an ENT doctor, the ENT doctor will be left with a bad impression of the dentist and his qualification as a professional dentist will be called into question. Therefore, it is important to master the indications for safe and reliable application of the osteotome technique.

> **! Key Point**
>
> If primary implant stability cannot be attained, the surgery should be discontinued.

### Clinical report 5A: Dislocation of an implant into the maxillary sinus

This patient visited our clinic with a loose implant inside the maxillary sinus. The patient had received two implants in the posterior maxilla, but one of them (R1) dislocated into the maxillary sinus and the patient was referred to us. The R1 implant had been placed using the osteotome technique 3 weeks ago and the patient complained of dull pain in the right cheek.

On the panoramic radiograph taken during the first visit, an implant was detected at region 16 that

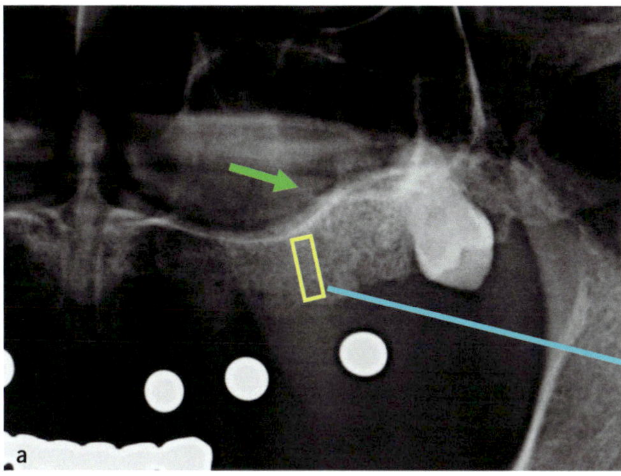

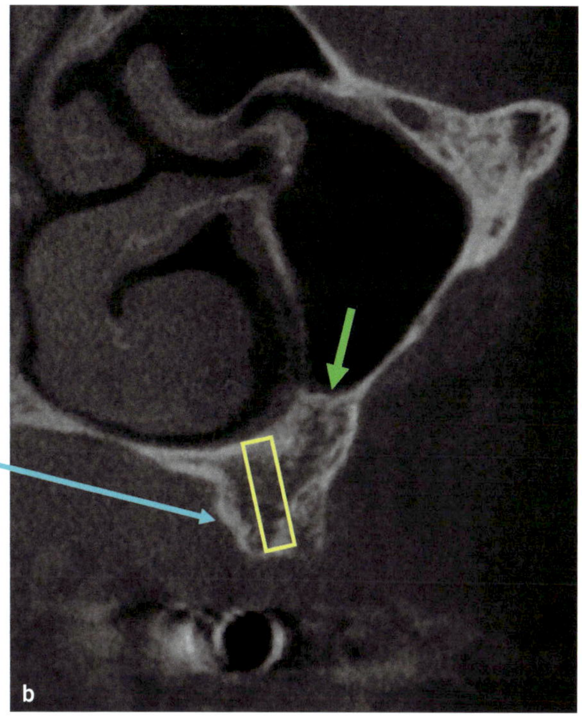

**Fig 6-14** (a and b) Panoramic view and CT image obtained during treatment planning.

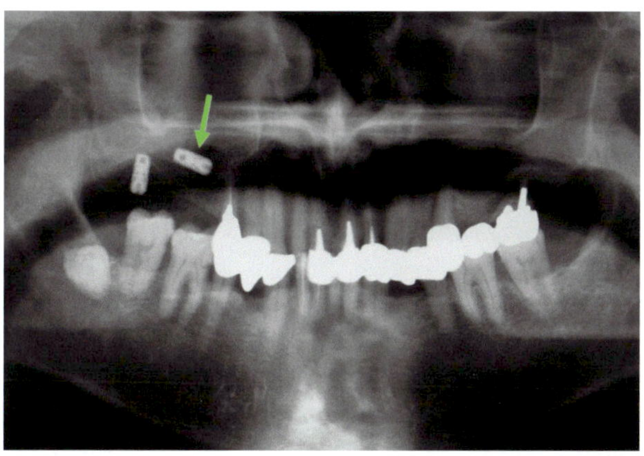

**Fig 6-15** Panoramic view on presentation.

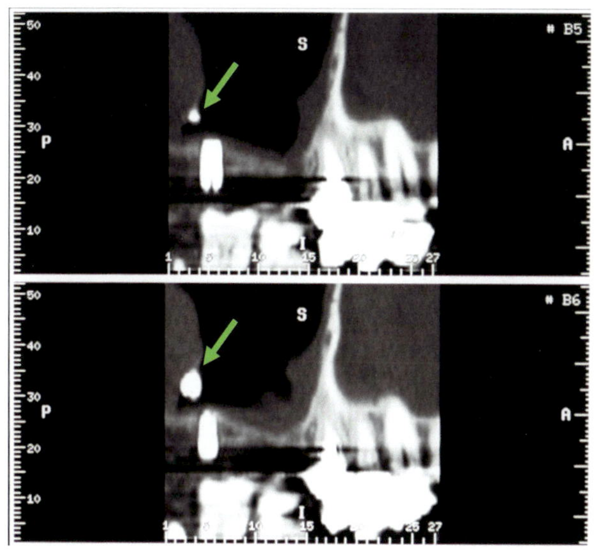

**Fig 6-16** Helical CT images on presentation.

had dislocated into the maxillary sinus (green arrow on Fig 6-15).

In addition, on the same visit, swelling of the maxillary sinus membrane was observed on the helical CT image, and R1 was present in the posterior of R2 (green arrows on Fig 6-16). Panoramic radiography was performed in the upright position, whereas the helical CT scan was performed in a supine position. The implant located at region 16 in the upright position moved to the back of R2 in the supine position. Based on these findings, the implant was considered to have become completely detached (Fig 6-17).

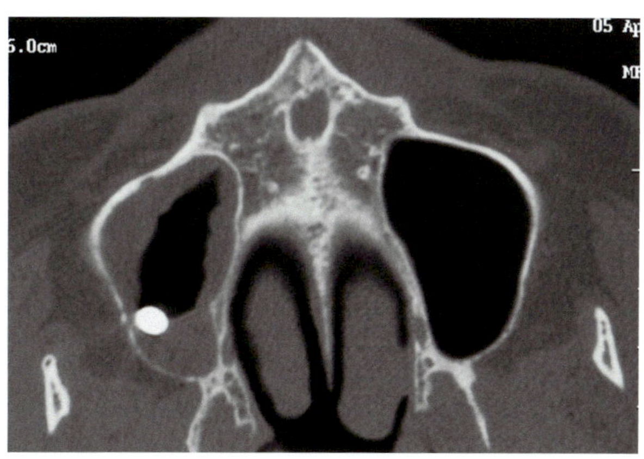

**Fig 6-17** CT image on presentation.

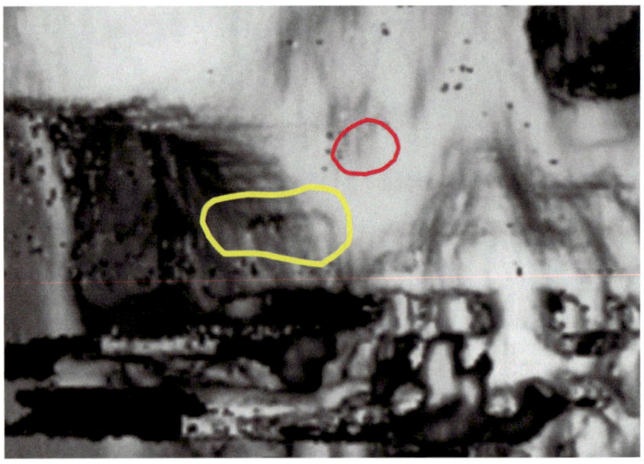

**Fig 6-18** An approach taking into consideration the sinus floor elevation and implant position (yellow line – osteotomy for sinus floor elevation in future; red line – current osteotomy).

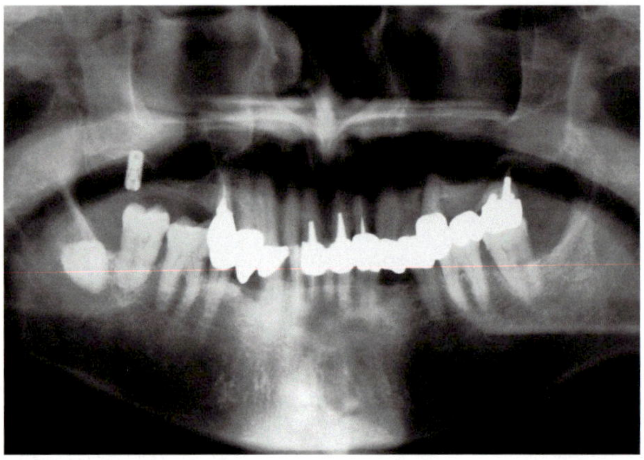

**Fig 6-19** Panoramic view after removal of the dislocated implant.

To replace an implant, sinus floor elevation is considered necessary. Approach from the canine fossa is considered optimal to prevent damage to the maxillary sinus anterior wall (Fig 6-18). Taking into account that the implant will be removed in a supine position, the implant is expected to have moved to the posterior wall of the sinus. Even if drilling is made at region 16, the implant will not be there!

Using intravenous sedation, the surgery for implant removal was performed under local anesthesia. The dislocated implant was present at the posterior wall of the maxillary sinus. White debris, which was believed to be a clump of bacteria, was found on the surface of the implant. The dislocated implant was easily removed using forceps for otological surgery (Fig 6-19).

## Clinical report 5B: Dislocation of an implant into the maxillary sinus

This case is an example of implant dislocation caused by a combination of poor primary stability, perforation of the sinus membrane, and postoperative swelling of the sinus membrane.

According to the patient's history, an implant had been placed at region 17 using the osteotome technique about 5 months earlier. The patient provided us with a panoramic radiograph taken immediately after the primary surgery, and this showed a dome-shaped bone-substitute–like radiopacity around the implant (yellow arrows on Fig 6-20a). Implant dislocation into the sinus cavity was found on the panoramic radiograph prior to the second surgery (green arrow on Fig 6-20b).

CT scanning at the patient's first visit to our clinic indicated a marked swelling of the sinus membrane and a dislocated implant inside the sinus cavity (Fig 6-21). A radiopacity was found at the implant socket (blue arrows on Fig 6-21a and b), which indicated that the healing of bone at the implant socket had already been completed.

The patient reported symptoms of sinusitis, such as dull pain in the buccal region on the right side and heaviness of the head, for about 1 month after implant surgery. These symptoms had been alleviated by continuous administration of medications. All these findings demonstrated the possibility that the implant dislocation into the sinus cavity had occurred shortly following the primary surgery. However, the question remained as to why the implant had dislocated, especially since it occurred against the force of gravity.

**! Key Point**

The force that pushes the implant up into the sinus cavity against the force of gravity is believed to be generated by the postoperative swelling of the sinus membrane that develops 1 week after surgery.

The author's speculations are as described below:

1. The implant was placed with the osteotome technique using bone substitutes, but failed to attain good primary stability.
2. During implant insertion, a perforation, which was too small to allow for leakage of the bone substitute into the sinus cavity occurred in the sinus membrane.
3. The mechanical stimulation from sinus membrane reflection induced swelling of the membrane 1 week after surgery. The swelling produced pressure,

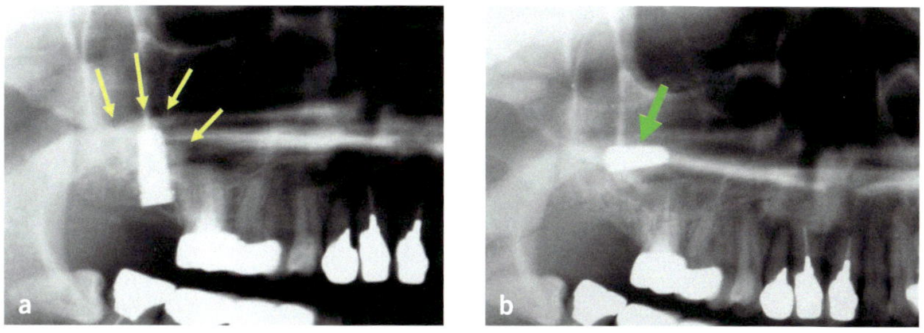

Fig 6-20 Panoramic views: (a) immediately after the primary surgery, provided by the patient; (b) new image on referral, about 5 months later.

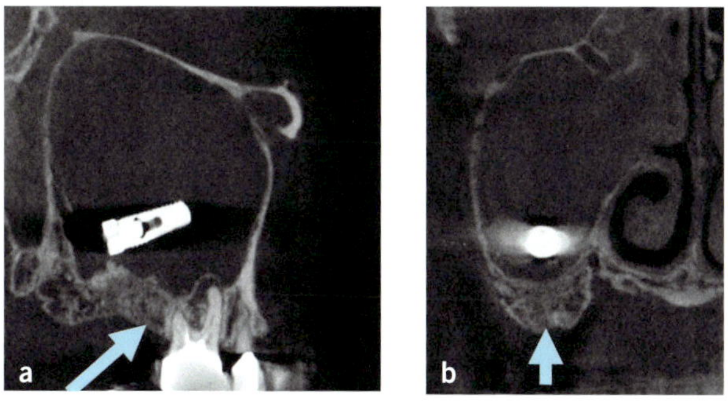

Fig 6-21 (a and b) CT images at the first visit.

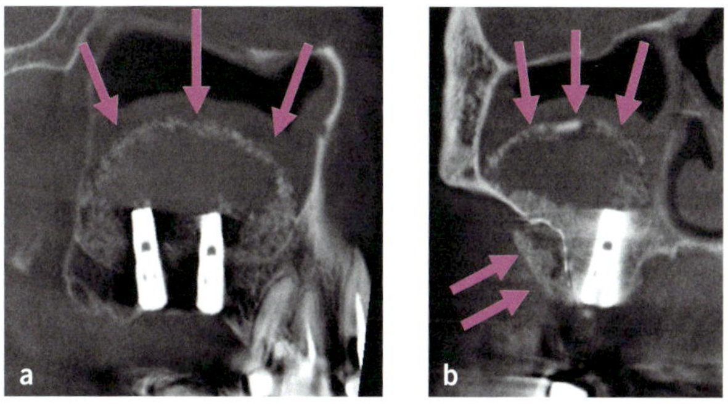

Fig 6-22 (a and b) CT images showing swelling of the sinus membrane occurring 1 week after sinus floor elevation.

not in one particular direction but in every direction, akin to an "explosion." The uppermost beta-tricalcium phosphate (β-TCP) granules were pushed up by this explosive pressure (pink arrows on Fig 6-22).

4. The postoperative swelling appears to have generated sufficient force to push and dislocate the implant upwards.
5. The bone substitute granules and the implant dislocated through the membrane perforation into the sinus cavity, resulting in maxillary sinusitis.
6. The dislocated bone substitute was gradually discharged through the ostium, which was the reason why the acute symptoms decreased within 1 month after the primary surgery.
7. Within the period of 5 months after primary surgery, the implant socket was filled with regenerated bone, whereas the implant dislocation inside the sinus cavity and the chronic maxillary sinusitis persisted as complications.

To minimize discomfort to the patient, surgery to remove the dislocated implant was performed under local anesthesia with intraveneous sedation. To approach through the sinus cavity, a hole was drilled through the bone at the canine fossa. The edematous maxillary sinus membrane was partially resected for better observation through the fiberscope. The dislocated implant was located inside the sinus cavity (Figs 6-23a and b). It was difficult to pick up the implant with the fiberscope probe and the implant was inadvertently pushed back even further into the posterior area.

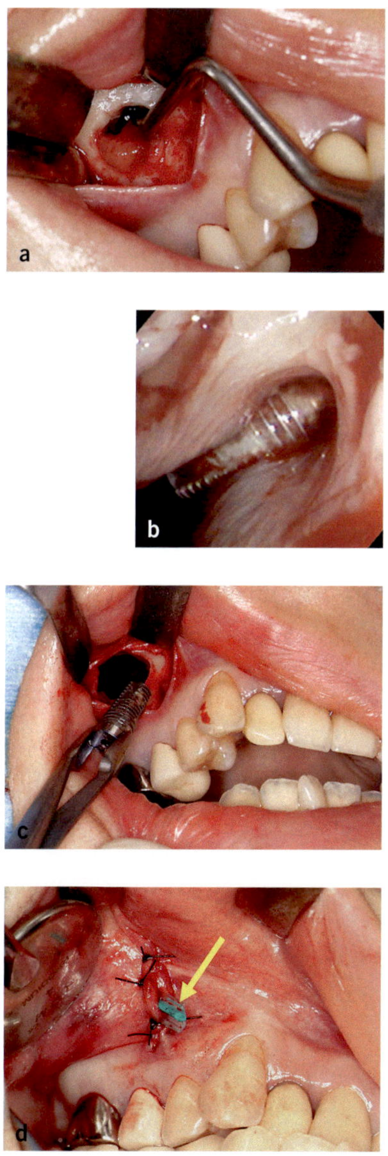

Fig 6-23 (a to d) Intraoperative intraoral views.

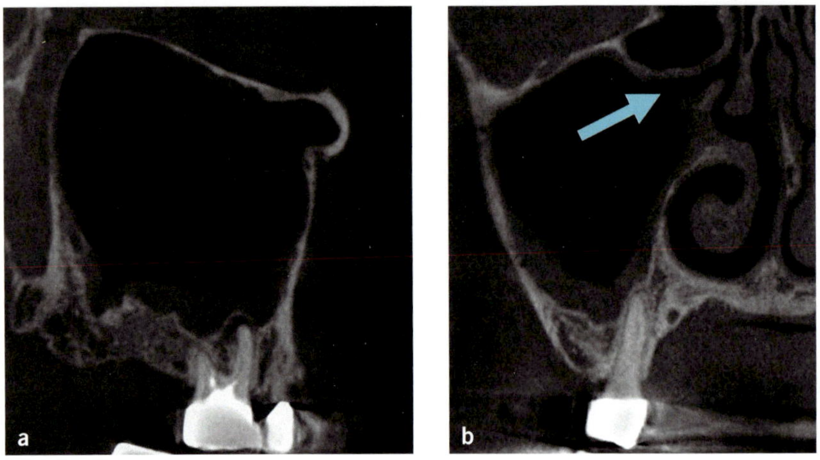

Fig 6-24 (a and b) Postoperative CT images.

> **! Key Point**
>
> Remove the dislocated implant using a fiberscope.

When monitoring through the fiberscope, the implant appeared to be located deep within the posterior region. Fortunately, the implant turned out to be located less deeply than expected, and it was removed easily with the forceps (Fig 6-23c). A drain was installed through the incision (yellow arrow on Fig 6-23d), and the wound was closed. Postoperative healing was uneventful.

A CT image obtained 3 months after the implant removal showed that membrane swelling had decreased and the opening of the ostium was intact (blue arrow on Fig 6-24d).

## Assessing implant osseointegration

Simultaneous implant placement with the osteotome technique cannot provide any assurance of osseointegration within the augmented site. Neither radiography nor CT scanning can prove successful osseointegration. The only way to evaluate the postoperative outcome is to indirectly estimate the osseointegration through the analysis, on CT images, of bone remodeling in the augmented area and the condition of the maxillary sinus membrane. If a given CT image shows no radiopacity in the augmented area and there is swelling of the sinus membrane, that should be interpreted as osseointegration failure.

### Clinical report 6A: Example of difficulties arising from simultaneous implant placement

This patient had experienced dislocation of implant R4 into the maxillary sinus during second surgery of R2, R3 and R4 and was referred to us. The implants R3 and R4 had been placed simultaneously with the osteotome technique. The R4 implant, from which the cover screw had already been removed, was found inside the maxillary sinus on the panoramic radiograph (yellow arrow on Fig 6-25). As shown on the intraoral view obtained during the first visit, the implants R2 and R3 and tooth 15 had been restored with provisional crowns (Fig 6-26). The buccolingual CT image at the first visit showed the dislocated implant R4 above implant R2 and swelling of the sinus membrane (Fig 6-27a). In addition, the superior alveolar artery was running along the anterior wall of the sinus (red arrow on Fig 6-27a). An abutment had been connected to the implant R3, but the apex of implant R3 appeared to penetrate into the maxillary sinus cavity (Fig 6-27b).

The dislocated implant was removed using a pair of tweezers through the hole drilled in the canine fossa (Figs 6-28a and b). Bleeding occurred from the superior alveolar artery during the drilling, which was arrested using an electric scalpel (blue arrow on Fig 6-28c). On the postoperative panoramic radiograph there is no R4 implant but the drain installed through the incision can be seen (yellow arrow on Fig 6-28d).

After removal of R4, a splinted superstructure was seated on R2, tooth 15 and R3 by the patient's regular dentist. The follow-up panoramic radiograph and buccolingual CT image taken at our clinic, however, revealed a sinking of R3 (yellow arrows on

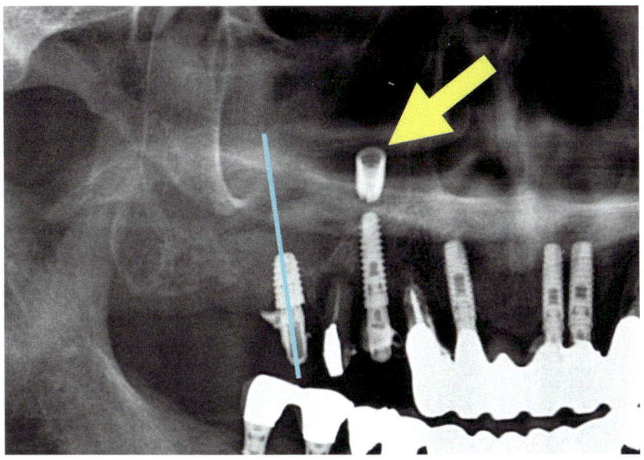

Fig 6-25 Panoramic view on referral.

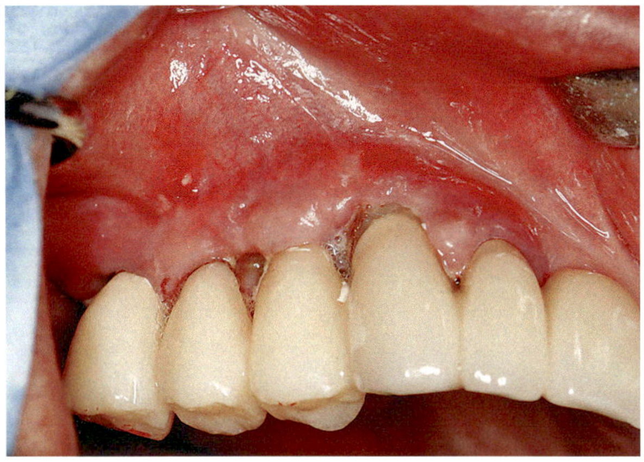

Fig 6-26 Intraoral view on referral.

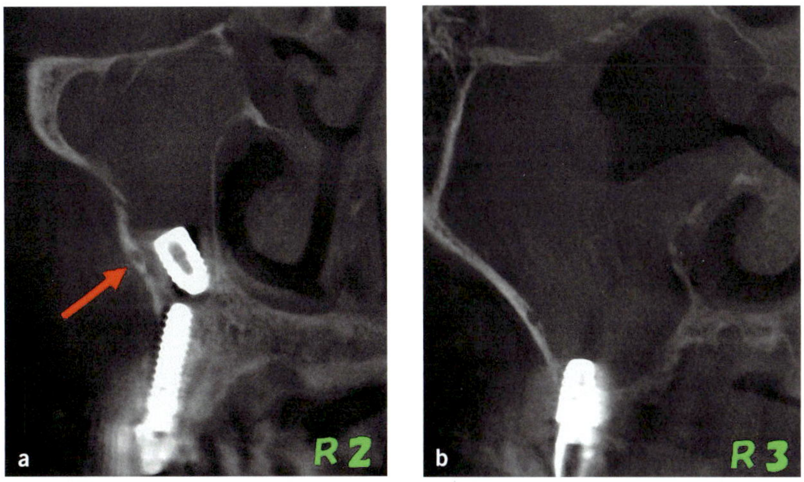


**Fig 6-27** (a and b) Buccolingual CT images at the first visit.

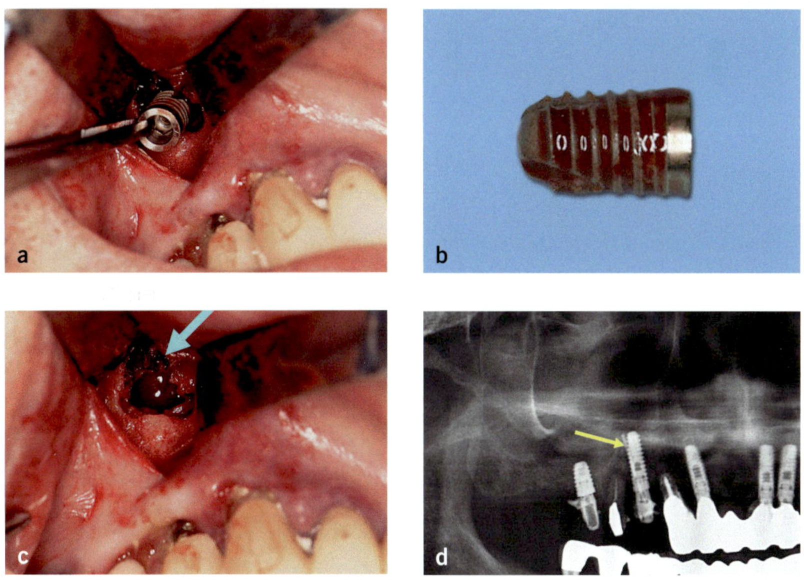


**Fig 6-28** (a to c) Intraoperative images; (d) panoramic view after the surgery.

Figs 6-29a and b) and residual swelling of the sinus membrane (Fig 6-29b).

Tooth 15 was judged hopeless and the splinted superstructure was split off between R2 and tooth 15, during which the crown on R2 detached together with the abutment (Figs 6-30a and b). Though the R2 implant maintained osseointegration, R3 presented with a lack of osseointegration and was removed together with tooth 15 as one block (Fig 6-30b). The fracture of the abutment screw of R2 was considered to have been caused by an excessive load on R2 induced by the mobility of tooth 15 and R3.

The patient's regular dentist reported that R3 was undergoing successful osseointegration at the

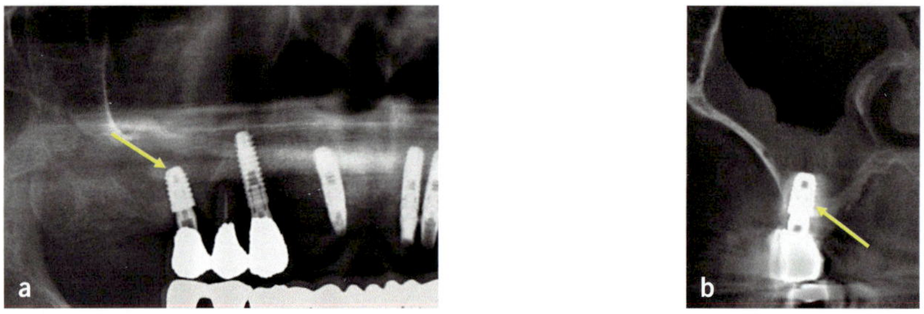

**Fig 6-29** Images obtained after remedial treatment by the patient's dentist: (a) panoramic view; (b) buccolingual CT image.

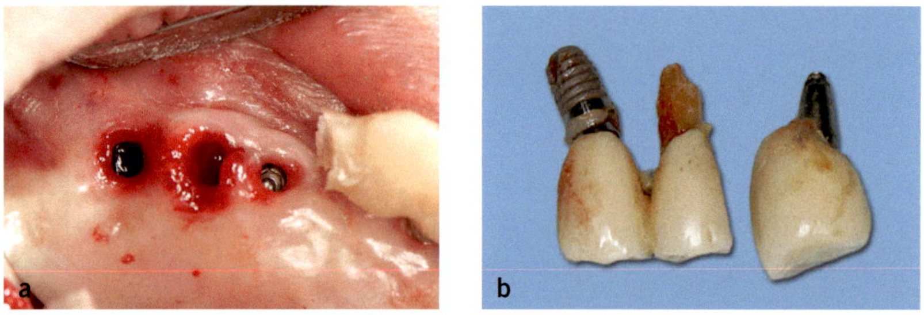

**Fig 6-30** (a and b) Removal of tooth 15 and implants.

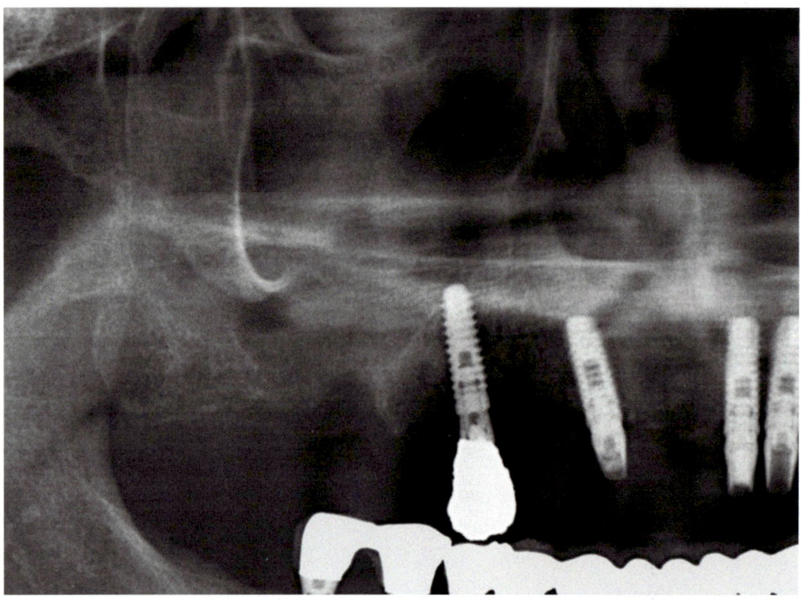

**Fig 6-31** Panoramic view after restoration of R2.

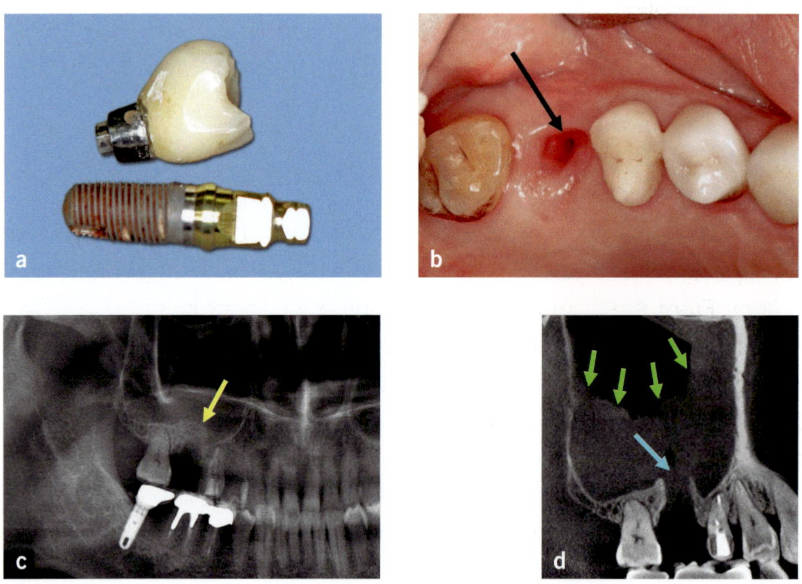

**Fig 6-32** Images at the first visit: (a) detached implant; (b) intraoral view; (c) panoramic view; (d) sagittal CT scan.

time of the second surgery. The osseointegration, however, was considered to have been limited only in the area of the residual bone. It is estimated that the absence of osseointegration in the augmented area led to the destruction of the osseointegration with the residual bone when it was subjected to a load.

The implant R2 was restored again with a new crown, but the implants R3 and R4, which had been placed simultaneously with the osteotome technique, were removed (Fig 6-31). In the case of this patient, re-treatment of the posterior maxilla on the right side by dental implants required sinus floor elevation by the lateral window technique. This involves waiting for bone healing in the implant socket and alleviation of the swelling of the sinus membrane.

> **! Key Point**
>
> For the next sinus floor elevation, we must wait for bone healing in the implant socket and alleviation of swelling of the sinus membrane, which means a significant extension of the entire treatment period and increased burden on the patient.

## Clinical report 6B: Uncertainty over the long-term prognosis

This patient was referred with the chief complaint of the loss of an implant placed 3 years earlier at region 16, with simultaneous application of the osteotome technique (Fig 6-32a). The patient was himself a dentist and brought a photo of the detached implant with him to the initial visit. There was dull pain in the buccal region on the right side, an oroantral fistula at region 16 (black arrow on Fig 6-32b), and air leakage through the nasal cavity when under positive intraoral pressure. A panoramic radiograph indicated a convex radiopacity in the upper area of region 16 (yellow arrow on Fig 6-32c), and it appears that bony tissue is present on the sinus floor. From the sagittal CT scan obtained during the first visit, however, no bony sinus floor above the implant socket was observed (blue arrow on Fig 6-32d), and there was swelling to the sinus membrane (green arrows on Fig 6-32d). Further, the implant socket wall was smooth, which indicates that the osseointegration had been lost for quite some time.

Based on the fact that the superstructure was connected, the implant was considered to have possessed osseointegration for a certain period. On the other hand, no bone can be seen at the sinus floor of the augmented site on the CT image taken during the first visit, so it appears unlikely that osseointegration had been achieved in the augmented site. Therefore, it was estimated that the implants were retained by the osseointegration only with the residual bone and that the occlusal load destroyed the limited osseointegration, resulting in the spontaneous implant detachment after several years of functional use.

As described in clinical report 6A above, there is no assurance that the implant inside the augmented site will achieve osseointegration. Therefore, there is a certain limitation in applying the osteotome technique to a single-stand implant. The author believes that, if the residual bone height is limited (1–6 mm), implants should be placed in a staged approach after sinus floor elevation by the lateral window technique.

> **! Key Point**
>
> It may appear that bony tissue is present on the sinus floor on a panoramic radiograph, whereas a CT scan demonstrates otherwise. A marked swelling of the maxillary sinus membrane is also precisely detected on a CT image.

Surgery to close the oroantral fistula was performed after the removal of soft tissue from the implant socket (Figs 6-33a–c). Healing of the soft tissue was adequate 3 months after surgery, and the oroantral fistula had disappeared (Fig 6-33d).

> **! Key Point**
>
> Close an oroantral fistula!

A decrease in the swelling of the sinus membrane was observed on the sagittal CT image obtained 1 month after this surgery (red arrows on Fig 6-34a). Three months following surgery, the membrane swelling had disappeared and the radiopacity at the bone defect had increased in density. The shape of the radiopacity around the implant socket differed from that observed before surgery, and the radiopaque line of the newly formed sinus floor was observed (Fig 6-34b). The line of the newly formed

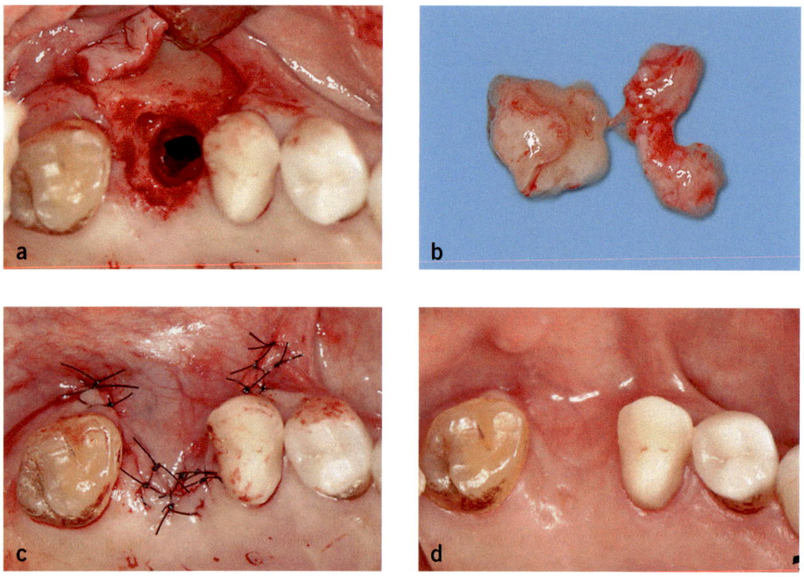

Fig 6-33 Surgery to close the oroantral fistula: (a to c) during the operation; (d) 3 months later.

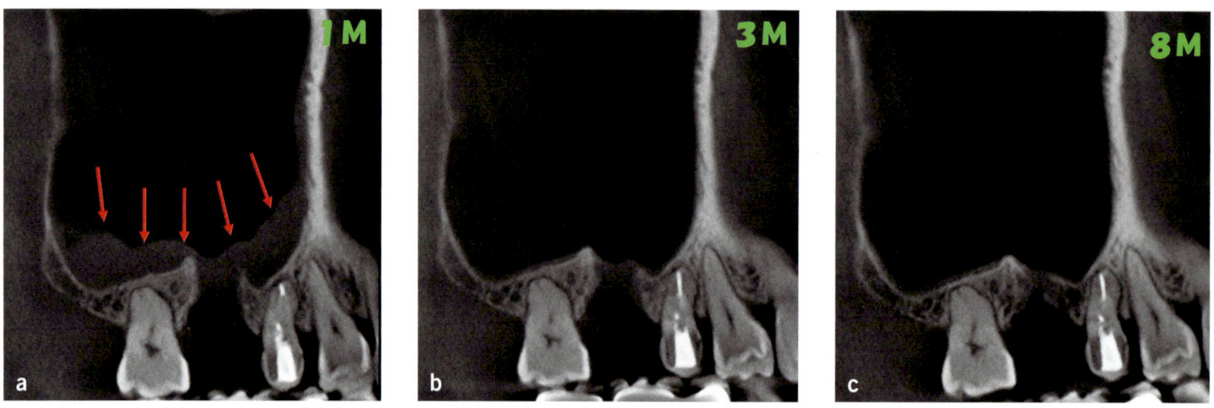


Fig 6-34 CT images after the closure: (a) at 1 month; (b) at 3 months; (c) at 8 months.

sinus floor was much more defined 8 months after surgery (Fig 6-34c). However, the recession at the ridge crest was significant and guided bone regeneration (GBR) was considered necessary.

Loss of osseointegration after implant restoration not only causes emotional stress to the patient but also requires a fairly difficult recovery procedure.

**! Key Point**

When the residual bone volume is limited, the maintenance of osseointegration remains questionable. Therefore, the indications for using the osteotome technique should be reviewed by accumulating reliable clinical data.